READING, WRITING AND DYSLEXIA: A COGNITIVE ANALYSIS

ANDREW W. ELLIS
Department of Psychology
University of Lancaster,
Lancaster, UK

LEA LAWRENCE ERLBAUM ASSOCIATES, PUBLISHERS LEA
London   Hillsdale, New Jersey

Lawrence Erlbaum Associates, Ltd., Publishers
Chancery House
319 City Road
London EC1V 1LJ

British Library Cataloguing in Publication Data

Ellis, Andrew W.
   Reading, writing and dyslexia.
   1. Dyslexia   2. Reading—Remedial education
   i. Title
   371.91 '4   LB1050.5

   ISBN 0-86377-002-9
   ISBN 0-86377-003-7 pbk

Printed and bound in Great Britain by A. Wheaton & Co., Ltd., Exeter

For my mother and father

Contents

Preface

Reading and writing have been the objects of intensive psychological research in recent years. Much of this work has focused on the skilled reader and writer, but there have been other valuable and interesting approaches. One of these has been the analysis of how brain injury can impair reading and writing in previously literate adults—the study, that is, of the acquired dyslexias and dysgraphias. Developmental problems in learning to read and write have also been investigated by cognitive psychologists, as has the acquisition of literacy by normal children. It is my personal belief that real advances are being made on all these fronts, and this book is an attempt to summarize and convey those advances. The book is aimed primarily at students of psychology or education, but I have tried at the same time to make the book intelligible to parents, teachers, and anyone else coming afresh to the investigation of reading, writing, and dyslexia. In addition, the book contains accounts of much recent or unpublished research, and also some of my own ideas. I hope that on these grounds it will also interest professionals in the field.

Two people have had a particularly strong influence on the development of my own thinking about reading, writing, and dyslexia. They are John Marshall and John Morton, and I should like to take this opportunity to thank them publicly. I have been fortunate enough to have worked for the past five years at Lancaster University. I should like to thank all my colleagues for creating such a friendly and stimulating atmosphere, but I have benefited particularly from exchanges of ideas with Alan Collins, Lesley Galpin, Dennis Hay, Phil Levy, Diane Miller, Peter Morris, Mary Smyth, and, last only on alphabetic grounds, Andy Young. If this book has any merit whatsoever it is due in no small measure to the extremely helpful comments on earlier drafts received from Max Coltheart, Karalyn Patterson, Leslie Henderson, Alan Collins, Tim Miles, and Maggie Snowling. I only wish I could have answered satisfactorily all of the points they raised. Alan Collins prepared the indices, Anne Parker, Sylvia Sumner, and Hazel Satterthwaite typed various portions of various drafts, and Anne Jackson drew the figures. My thanks to them. The writing of this book was facilitated by grants HR 7485 and CO 023-2042 from the Social Science Research Council.

Finally I should like to thank Anna for everything, and Martin and Hayden for helping me maintain a sense of proportion.

Andrew W. Ellis
Lancaster, April 1983

Introduction

Reading has always occupied a central place within the branch of psychology known as "cognitive psychology," and it still continues to hold that position. Cognitive psychologists are interested in understanding the nature and organization of the many psychological processes which make reading and writing possible. They are interested in such things as how we identify letters and words, how we comprehend sentences and texts, how we are able to pronounce both familiar and unfamiliar words, how we know what sequence of letters to use when we wish to write a word, and so on. The general approach is commonly known as "information processing": it regards reading and writing as skills made possible by the concerted activity of many component processes whose workings it is the job of cognitive psychologists to unravel.

The traditional research tool of the cognitive psychologist has been the controlled experiment, and this book makes use of the many insights gained from such experiments. However, particularly in recent years, psychologists have sought to advance our understanding by studying how brain injury may affect reading and/or writing in previously literate adults. It has been discovered that there are many forms of "acquired dyslexia" and "acquired dysgraphia" each caused by damage to different sets of cognitive processes. In general, less attention has been given to how children learn to read and write, and to the developmental disorders associated with the acquisition of literacy, but there are signs that even these areas are gradually yielding up their secrets to cognitive interrogation.

One of the difficulties in teaching the psychology of reading and writing is to get students to appreciate that there *are* problems here to be solved, and to understand what those problems are. Another difficulty lies in introducing the small amount of essential linguistic and psychological terminology in a nonfrightening way. I have found that a potted history of how writing has evolved, together with a brief inspection of the present-day English writing system, are a useful way of overcoming both these obstacles while retaining the student's interest. Chapter 1 is, therefore, given over to just such a potted history and brief inspection. Chapters 2 and 3 gradually build up a model of how skilled readers identify, comprehend, and pronounce printed words. Chapter 4 discusses how brain injury can disrupt these same operations and considers what the observed patterns of breakdown can tell us about the nature of normal, intact reading processes. Chapter 5 tackles the reading and comprehension of sentences and texts by skilled readers, while Chapter 6 looks at the production of written language—at writing, spelling, and the acquired dysgraphias. By Chapter 7 we are ready to examine how normal children learn to read and write. Finally, Chapter 8 considers the somewhat controversial topic of developmental dyslexia and advocates an approach similar to that which has proved so successful in analyzing the acquired dyslexias and dysgraphias.

1 Written Language

When we say that a child has learned to read we mean that he or she is able both to understand and to pronounce written language. In the vast majority of cases this follows an earlier mastery of spoken language. Simple observations like these mean that it will help us to understand both reading and writing if we first examine written language and consider how it relates to spoken language.

THE ORIGINS OF WRITING

Prehistoric people used pictures to convey information, as did (or do) several recent cultures without writing systems in North America, Central Africa, Southeastern Asia, and Siberia. Figure 1.1 shows a rock drawing found near a precipitous trail in New Mexico. It warns the "reader" that, while a mountain goat (with horns) may hope to pass safely, a rider on horseback is certain to fall. "Picture writing" of this sort may be quite sophisticated in what it conveys. Figure 1.2 shows a drawing found on the face of a rock in Michigan on the shore of Lake Superior and relates the course of an Indian military expedition.

The meaning of the drawing is provided by Gelb (1962, pp. 29–30). The five canoes at the top carry fifty-one men, represented by the vertical strokes. A chieftain called Kishkemunasee, "Kingfisher," leads the expedition. He is represented by the bird drawn above the first canoe. The

1

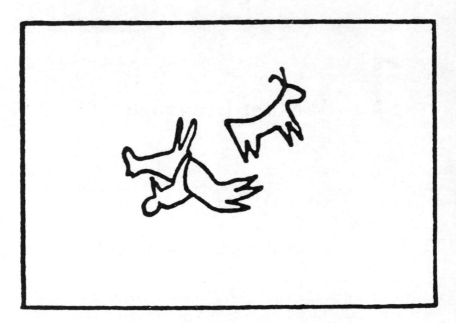

Figure 1.1   Indian rock drawing from New Mexico (from G. Mallery, *Picture-Writing of the American Indians*. Tenth Annual Report of the Bureau of Ethology, Smithsonian Institution, Washington, 1893).

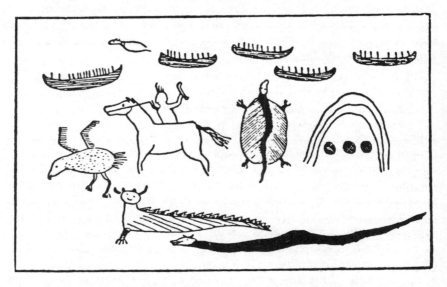

Figure 1.2   Indian rock drawing from Michigan (from H. R. Schoolcraft, *Historical and Statistical Information, Respecting the History, Condition, and Prospects of the Indian Tribes of the United States*, Part 1, Philadelphia, 1851).

three suns under three arches show that the journey lasted three days. The turtle symbolizes a happy landing, and the picture of a man on a horse shows that the warriors marched on quickly. The courageous spirit of the warriors is captured in the drawing of the eagle, while force and cunning are evoked in the symbols of the panther and serpent.

Two points can be made. First, the interpretation of Figure 1.2, like the interpretation of some of our traffic signs, is by no means self-evident: one needs to be a member of the culture to know, for example, that a turtle can symbolize a happy landing. The second point is that there is no one, correct way to "read" Figure 1.2; its meaning may be expressed many ways in English and no doubt in equally many ways in the language of the North American Indian who drew it.

THE EMERGENCE OF TRUE WRITING

Historical evidence suggests that "picture writing" of the sort just illustrated gradually became more formal and more abstract (see Diringer, 1962; Gelb, 1963). A circle, formerly used to represent the sun, could also be used to mean "heat," "light," "day," or a god associated with the sun. Such stylized picture writing is known as "ideographic writing," but it remains the case that a message in ideographic writing can be "read" in a wide variety of ways. True writing systems emerged for the first time when writing symbols were used to represent *words of the language* rather than objects or concepts. The important step has probably been taken independently in a number of places at different times.

The earliest true writing systems are based, then, on the one-word-one-symbol principle. Such writing systems are called "logographic" (from the Greek word *logos* meaning word), and individual symbols are known as "logograms." Modern Chinese is still logographic, as is one of the writing systems (*Kanji*) used in Japan (see Figure 1.3). In time the logograms of the early writing systems such as Sumerian cuneiform and Egyptian hieroglyphics became progressively less picture like. Such increasing arbitrariness may have fostered a change of attitude whereby logograms ceased to be considered as directly (or solely) representing *meanings* and came to be regarded as representing *words*. When this happens, a logogram may be used not only for its original meaning but also for a word with the same *sound* (as if a circle meaning "sun" were also used to represent the word "son" or, to borrow an example from Fromkin and Rodman (1974), as if two logograms for "bee" and " leaf" were combined to represent the abstract word "belief").

This progression toward using logograms to represent word-sounds occurred with Egyptian hieroglyphics and was further developed when the

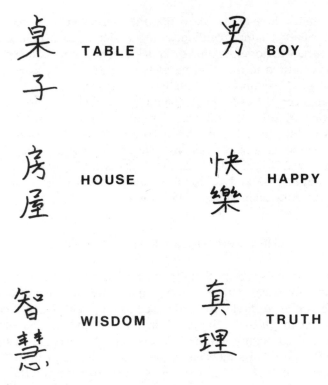

Figure 1.3 Examples of Chinese logographs.

Egyptian symbols were borrowed by a people who lived on the eastern shores of the Mediterranean—the Phoenecians. They spoke an entirely different language from the Egyptians but used the hieroglyphic symbols to represent the *syllables* of their own language. In the hands of the Phoenecians, then, the conversion of Egyptian hieroglyphs from a logographic system to a *syllabic system* was completed (around 1500 BC). The progression toward the representation of sounds in writing took a further step with the invention of the *alphabet*. Many writing systems in use today, including our own, are alphabets. As a first approximation (which will be qualified later) we can say that an alphabet employs a different letter, or a group of letters, for each sound in the spoken language. This may seem like a simple and natural way to organize a writing system, but in fact the alphabetic principle has been discovered only once—by the Greeks around 1000 BC. The Greeks borrowed the syllabic Phoenecian writing system but adapted it by using a different written character for each of the different consonant and vowel sounds of their spoken language. All modern alphabets are descendents of the Greek version (ours comes via the Roman alphabet).

THE ORIGINS OF ENGLISH SPELLING

In what we might call a "transparent" alphabetic writing system the spelling of each word would convey that word's pronunciation clearly and unambiguously. Some modern alphabets, such as Finnish, Italian, and Latvian come close to being transparent in this way. English written words like *dog*, *ship*, and *pistol* are also transparent (or "regular") because their pronunciation is straightforwardly predictable to anyone who knows the normal correspondences between English letters and sounds. However, as teachers are only too well aware, many written English words deviously conceal their pronunciations. One need only contemplate such opaque "irregular" or "exception" words as *women, yacht, debt, island, knight,* and *colonel* to appreciate the truth of this.

Interestingly, English has not always contained the sorts of irregularly spelled words we find in today's books. Before about 1500 AD English words were spelled as they were pronounced, which means that spellings varied from place to place as their dialect pronunciations varied. According to Stubbs (1980) the first irregularities were introduced into English by professional scribes who disliked the confusing repetition of up-down strokes in words like *wimin, munk,* and *wunder*. (Try writing *aluminum* in rapid, cursive writing and you will appreciate the problem.) To facilitate rapid writing the scribes changed the spellings to *women, monk,* and *wonder* thereby creating the first irregular English words. More followed after William Caxton established the first printing press in England. The spread and development of printing brought with it a gradual standardization of spellings which ceased to reflect regional variations in pronunciation. Many early printers were Dutch and unsure of how English speakers pronounced certain words; it was they who put the *ch* in *yacht* because the equivalent Dutch word contained a consonant similar to that in the Scottish pronunciation of the word *loch*.

To complicate matters further, there were at large in the fifteenth and sixteenth centuries influential spelling reformers. They differed from their present-day counterparts in that they wanted to alter spellings in such a way as to reflect the Latin or Greek origins of words at the expense of transparency. Thus *dette* became *debt, doute* became *doubt,* and *sutil* became *subtle* to reflect the historical origins of these words in the Latin words *debitum, dubite,* and *subtilis* respectively. Sometimes, alas, the reformers got it wrong. They introduced a *c* in *scissors* and *scythe* because they thought (wrongly) that both words derived from the Latin word *scindere* (to cleave); similarly we owe our modern spelling of *anchor* to a false historical link with the Greek word *anchorite*. Other examples of false etymology are the *s* in *island* (formerly *iland*) and the *h* on *hour* (*oure*); none of these letters have ever been pronounced in English.

English spellings were more or less fully standardized by 1650, and the process was completed by the production in the eighteenth century of the first dictionaries, the best known being Dr. Samuel Johnson's *Dictionary of the English Language* (1755). Indeed, according to Stubbs (1980) the concept of a "spelling error" hardly existed before about 1770—prior to that time if a spelling sounded right it *was* right.

Apart from occasional irregularities introduced by scribes, Dutch printers, or spelling reformers, the majority of spellings to be found in the great dictionaries accurately reflected contemporary pronunciations. However, pronunciations change while spellings, fossilized in the dictionaries, remain immutable. In the seventeenth century *knave* and *knife* were pronounced with a /k/, the /l/ was pronounced in *would* and *should*, and a sound like the *ch* in *loch*, and spelled *gh*, occurred in *right, light, bought, eight*, and similar words. As the pronunciation of all these words has changed over the last three hundred years, so their spellings, which were once regular and rational, have become irregular. Changes in pronunciation unaccompanied by changes in spelling are responsible for many of the irregularities in the spelling-sound correspondences of present-day English. Unlike the Dutch or the Germans we have never reformed our spellings to bring them back into line with changes in pronunciation.

One trend has attempted to restore spelling-sound correspondence in some measure. Until the late eighteenth century there was no *h* sound in the pronunciation of words like *habit, hotel, hospital, history*, and *herb*, but under the influence of spelling the *h* has been introduced in many dialects (exceptions being the refined pronunciation of *hotel* without an *h*, and those regional dialects whose speakers are accused of "dropping their aitches" but in fact never caught them in the first place). Other examples of pronunciation changing to accommodate to spelling are the switch from *t* to *th* in words like "anthem," "author," and "theatre," and the introduction of a *t* sound in the word *often*. Despite the oft-repeated claim by linguists that theirs is a "descriptive" rather than a "prescriptive" discipline, it is easy to detect a note of condescension in many treatments of spelling pronunciation. Such a patronizing attitude seems to be both inappropriate and unfair; spelling pronunciation can just as well be viewed as an effort after rationality on the part of native speakers faced with what can often seem (at first blush anyway) like a quite irrational orthography.

LEVELS OF REPRESENTATION IN PRESENT-DAY ENGLISH SPELLING

As we have seen, all writing systems began by using logographs with a different symbol for each word. Some, but not all, systems have evolved into alphabets with symbols for each distinctive sound. In the case of English spelling it is as if a tension has existed between the demand of an alphabet for transparency and a wish to retain something of the old logographic principle. In fact the situation is a little more complex than even that generalization suggests.

Spoken language is hierarchically structured in that sentences can be divided up into clauses, clauses into phrases, and phrases into words. Words can then be divided into smaller units of meaning called *morphemes*. The term "morpheme" is not familiar outside linguistics, but it is a useful and important one. A word like *trust* is a one-morpheme word, but *trustful* contains two morphemes, *trust* and *-ful*. *Distrustful* contains three morphemes, *dis-*, *trust*, and *-ful*, while *distrustfully* adds a fourth. These multi-morpheme words usually contain a "root morpheme" (*trust* in our example), plus one or more "bound morphemes" like *dis-*, *-ful*, *-ing*, *-s*, or *-ed* which never occur in isolation, and which in some way modify the meaning and/or the grammatical function of the root. Morphemes can, in turn, often be subdivided into distinctive sounds (or *phonemes*). Thus, *trust* contains one phoneme in its pronunciation for each letter in its spelling, though *cheat* contains five letters but only three phonemes represented by *ch*, *ea*, and *t*.

The English orthography tries in one way or another to represent in print each of these units or levels of the spoken language. Sentences are marked by initial capital letters and terminal full stops (or periods). Commas, semi-colons, and colons can be used to mark off clauses and phrases, while words are separated by spaces.

The word level of representation

The influence of the word level on English spelling is felt in more ways than just the placing of spaces. Although English has a few logographs like &, $, and £, a more important logographic influence can be appreciated if we consider the irregular words *two*, *sword*, *hymn*, *damn*, and *sign*, and particularly if we pair them with the words *too*, *soared*, *him*, *dam*, and *sine*. The point is that these are all *homophones*—words which sound alike but have different meanings. It is possible for both alternative spellings of a word to be regular if there is more than one regular way of spelling a phoneme. This applies, for example, to *bean* and *been*, or *loot* and *lute*. For words like *him* and *dam*, however, any alternative must be irregular. One consequence of reforming spellings to permit only one way of representing each sound visually would be a loss of the present visual distinctions between many homophones.

Another word-level influence was noted by Chomsky and Halle (1968) in their book *The Sound Pattern of English* which modified many people's views on English spelling (see Halle, 1969; Chomsky, 1970 for reasonably accessible summaries). The influence in question can be discerned if we consider why the silent *g* might occur in *sign* and the silent *b* in *bomb*. As Chomsky and Halle noted, there are words related in meaning to *sign* and *bomb* in which these silent letters *are* pronounced—for example, *signature* and *bombard*. Removing the silent letters would result in a loss of the visual clues to relatedness of meaning between such words.

The morphemic level of representation

Dropping down a level from words to morphemes uncovers another form of representation in English spelling. In the written words *ropes*, *robes*, and *roses* the root morphemes *rope*, *robe*, and *rose* are modified by the addition of the plural morpheme represented by the letter *s*. Listen closely however to the spoken words *ropes*, *robes*, and *roses* and you will hear that the plural ending of *ropes* is "s," that the ending of *robes* is "z," and the the ending of *roses* is "iz." More accurate spellings from the alphabetic standpoint might be ROPES, ROBEZ, and ROSIZ, but such spellings would disguise the presence of the same plural morpheme at the end of each word.

In an experiment reported by Baker (1980), volunteer individuals (who in psychology are conventionally known as "subjects") were asked to pretend that they were either linguists trying to capture the pronunciation of words as accurately as possible in their spellings, or spelling reformers trying to produce rational, intelligent spellings. When being linguists the majority of subjects opted for the ROPES, ROBEZ, and ROSIZ types of spellings, whereas when the same individuals were being spelling reformers they opted to ignore differences in pronunciation and preserve the one-to-one correspondence between written -*s* and the plural morpheme; that is, to retain the existing spellings.

Another example of spellings preserving morphemic identity at the expense of alphabetic transparency concerns the spelling of the past tense morpheme in words like *flapped*, *soared*, and *glided*. A spelling reformer devoted to transparency might respell these FLAPT, SOARD, and GLIDID but in so doing he or she would lose the morphemic correspondence between written -*ed* and the past tense morpheme.

The phonemic level of representation

Although some writing systems such as Japanese *Kana* operate on a one symbol for each syllable basis, spoken English has too many different syllables for this principle to form the basis of our spelling, and syllabic representation occurs only in oddities like BAR-B-Q. To represent pronunciation English spelling utilizes the alphabetic principle of one letter (or a group of letters) for each sound.

In fact, it is not quite accurate to say that alphabetic symbols represent all the different *sounds* of the spoken language. The "p" sound in the spoken word "pit" is slightly, but perceptibly different from the "p" sound in "spit," the latter being less "aspirated." Similarly the "l" sound in "light" is different from the "l" in "dull." Our alphabet, however, ignores such minor differences and only has separate letters for sounds which distinguish words with different meanings. (The Russian language uses the two *l*'s mentioned above to distinguish different words and so has two different letters for them.) In linguistics the term *phoneme* is used for sounds which distinguish words with different meanings, so alphabetic spellings should really be described as employing distinct letters for different phonemes.

Regular, transparent English words like *dog* or *catamaran* employ one letter for each phoneme in the spoken form of the word. Sometimes two or more letters (or *graphemes*)[1] will correspond to a single phoneme—for example, the *ch* in *chip*, the *th* in *bath*, and the *oo* in *moon*. When a final *e* is used to change the middle vowel of *bit* to *bite* or *tap* to *tape*, then the rules necessary to translate spellings into pronunciations become still more complex. Further, some vowel sounds can be spelled in more than one regular way (compare *hEAt*, *strEEt* and *complEtE*). Some letter strings are given two different and inconsistent pronunciations in different sets of words (compare *mint* and *pint*), and so on.

The irregularities, inconsistencies, and multiple levels of correspondence in English spelling undoubtedly create problems for the learner. English spelling has been described as adapted to suit the needs of the already skilled reader and speller, and there is certainly an element of truth in that generalization. However, while being a nuisance for the learner, the vagaries of English spelling constitute a rich vein of material for the psychologist to exploit, which is one reason why we have devoted some time to analyzing them.

SUMMARY OF CHAPTER 1

Writing may be distinguished from other means of visual communication because in writing the symbols correspond to, or represent units of, the spoken language rather than directly expressing objects of concepts. The earliest writing systems employed a different symbol for each *word* in the

---

[1]Different authors use the term grapheme somewhat differently, Here *grapheme* and *letter* will be taken to be more or less synonymous and interchangeable.

TABLE 1.1
Levels of representation in present-day English spelling

LEVEL	EXAMPLES
1. WORD LEVEL	1(a) *logographs*: £ & $ + − %
	1(b) *distinguishing homophones*
	or—oar be—bee
	one—won two—too
	would—wood piece—peace
	rain—rein—reign
	peek—peak—pique
	1(c) *representing relatedness of meaning*
	sign—signature bomb—bombard
	nation—native damn—damnation
2. MORPHEME LEVEL	*Constant spellings of morphemes despite changes in pronunciation*
	soared—flapped—glided
	ropes—robes—roses
3. PHONEME LEVEL	*Phonemically transparent (alphabetic) spellings of regular words*
	bit—dull—melon—token
	divine—shack—market—pelvis

language. Since then, some writing systems have evolved ways of additionally representing smaller units of language (the *morpheme*, *syllable*, and *phoneme*).

English employs an *alphabet*—that is, a writing system which includes a level of correspondence between letters (graphemes) and phonemes. At the same time, however, English shows tendencies towards word-level correspondence; for example, in its small number of logographs (&, £, $, etc.) and, more importantly, in the visual differentiation of homophones like *plain* and *plane*. Morphemic influences show in the constant spelling of morphemes like the plural -*s* and the past tense -*ed* despite changes in pronunciation. Because of these and other factors, although many English spellings are transparent or *regular*, many others are opague or *irregular* in that their pronunciation cannot easily be deduced from their spelling. The various levels of representation incorporated into English spelling are shown in Table 1.1.

2   Reading by Ear and by Eye

The discussion of the English writing system in the previous chapter has hopefully equipped us to advance to asking the psychological question, "How do skilled readers recognize written words?" Our first task is to realize that there *is* a problem here to be solved. Reading comes so easily to the fluent reader that it is sometimes hard to appreciate the complexity of the psychological processes which permit this rather effortless performance. To an extent, being able to read is rather like being able to drive a car—you soon forget how hard it was to learn and, especially when things are going smoothly, you progress with scant regard for the machinery which makes the progression possible. And yet the machinery *is* there, and complicated machinery it is too, as one discovers when something *does* go wrong. So the ease of skilled reading should not blind us to the intricacy of the mental operations responsible for that performance. In this chapter we shall describe some of the processes which enable skilled readers to recognize written words. However, we shall begin by taking a step back and first considering how, as listeners, we are able to recognize and comprehend *spoken* words.

READING BY EAR

When someone speaks, the sound travels through the air to the listener as sound waves. Those waves strike the listener's ear and are converted by machinery inside the ear into a pattern of nervous impulses which travel along nerves to the brain. Each perceptibly different word will set up a different pattern of nerve impulses which may be thought of as an *acoustic code* specifying a word which the speaker has just produced. Identifying an acoustic code *x* as the code for word *y* is a problem of pattern recognition. This problem has been faced and partially solved by engineers and psychologists who have tried to build and program computers to understand speech. In systems such as the one described by Klatt (1981) the computer is equipped with an array of *auditory word recognition units*. Each unit responds to the sound wave characteristic of a different spoken word. So when a speaker addresses the computer by uttering a word into a microphone, each of the recognition units tests the input against its own specifications. The unit which makes the best match will be the most active, and the computer will operate on the assumption that the word represented by that unit was the one just uttered by the speaker.

These computer models may also provide useful analogies to help us think about human word recognition. Thus, many theories of human speech comprehension incorporate the notion of auditory word recognition units, one for each of the spoken words with which the listener is familiar (e.g., Morton, 1979a; Marslen-Wilson, 1982). It is sometimes helpful to represent such models or theories in terms of an "information-processing diagram" like the one shown in Figure 2.1. This figure is meant to represent the stages involved when we recognize and understand a word we hear spoken. First, the sound wave strikes our ears and is converted into an *acoustic code* by the *acoustic analysis system* of the ear and auditory portions of the brain. That acoustic code is transmitted to an *auditory word recognition system* where, if the code is one for a familiar word, it will activate its particular recognition unit. The listener then "hears" a particular word, and the appropriate meaning becomes available. In Figure 2.1 and all subsequent figures, the dotted line represents the boundary between the external, physical word and internal, psychological processes.

The relevance of all this to the psychology of reading can be appreciated if you try answering the following questions:

1 Is a PHOKS an animal?
2 Can you sail in a YOTT?
3 Should we build our HOWZIZ from straw?

Hopefully the reader will agree that the answers to these questions are "Yes," "Yes," and "Not if we wish to avoid being eaten by big bad wolves" respectively. How is it that strange and unfamiliar letter strings like PHOKS, YOTT, and HOWZIZ can be comprehended this way? Part of the answer must lie in the alphabetic aspect of English spelling. With-

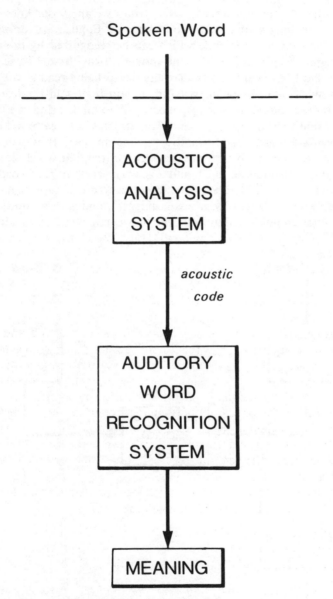

Figure 2.1 A simple information-processing diagram to represent some of the processes and stages involved in recognizing a heard word.

out ever having seen PHOKS before we can pronounce it to ourselves, knowing for example that PH at the beginning of a word is pronounced "f." In order to pronounce these letter strings we apply our knowledge of the regular spelling-sound correspondences of English. In doing so we create an *internal* acoustic code which can be recognized by the auditory word recognition system just as if the spoken words "fox," "yacht," and "houses" had been heard rather than the words being read in the form of these somewhat odd misspellings. (In fact, *yott* is the old English spelling of *yacht* before the word was respelled by the Dutch printers.)

These examples illustrate a mode or strategy of reading known as *phonic mediation* or, less formally, reading by ear. It is a strategy a reader can use when he or she encounters an unfamiliar word on a printed page—that is, "sound it out" and discover whether the word *sounds* familiar even when it doesn't *look* familiar. We can represent the processes involved in reading by ear as a diagram, and this is done in Figure 2.2. The first thing one must do with a written word is to identify its

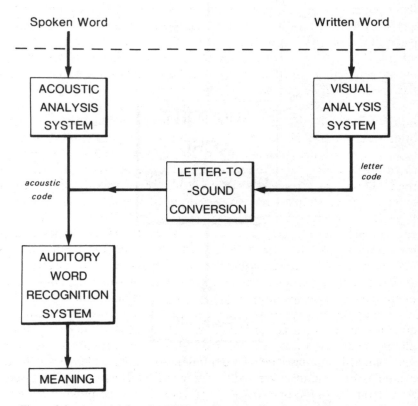

Figure 2.2 A model for phonically mediated reading, or "reading by ear."

component letters. With clear print this is no problem, but if one is reading ornate script or untidy handwriting letter identification can be far from easy. Just as a sound wave must first be analyzed by an acoustic analysis system, so a printed word must be analyzed by a *visual analysis system* whose job it is to identify letters and create an internal *letter code*. In the case of reading by ear, the letter code must then be translated by *letter-sound conversion processes* into an *acoustic code* which can be identified by the auditory word recognition system.

PHONIC MEDIATION THEORY AND SOME OBJECTIONS TO IT

There is no question but that readers *can* use phonic mediation to recognize written words. Occasionally, however, cognitive psychologists have made the more radical suggestion that phonic mediation may be obligatory and unavoidable even when a highly fluent reader is reading a word he or she has read countless times before. To the best of my knowledge this suggestion was first made by the nineteenth-century German neurologist Carl Wernicke (1874), and it has been reiterated more recently by Rubenstein, Lewis, and Rubenstein (1971) and Gough (1972) among others. There are, however, a number of reasons why the theory of obligatory phonic mediation cannot be right (see Coltheart, 1980a; Patterson, 1982; Henderson, 1982 for recent reviews).

One line of evidence against phonic mediation theory comes from studies of "acquired dyslexia"; that is, from studies of the way injury to the brain (most commonly caused by a stroke) can disrupt reading in individuals who were once skilled readers. Now, as we shall see in Chapter 4, there are a variety of different acquired dyslexic syndromes. In one of these, known as "phonological dyslexia," patients are unable to read aloud even the simplest nonword such as PIB or ZUG. They appear to have lost the capacity for even the most rudimentary letter-to-sound conversion, and yet they are capable of both understanding and pronouncing almost any familiar real word (Patterson, 1982; Funnell, 1983). This must imply a psychological "route" from print to meaning which does *not* depend on letter-sound conversion and which remains intact in phonological dyslexics despite damage to the phonic route.

Although neuropsychological evidence of the sort just discussed is valuable, it may not be necessary to go to such lengths in order to realize that phonic mediation theory faces some rather grave difficulties. As we have seen, English contains many homophones—words which have different meanings but sound alike. Now, if a word's meaning were accessed entirely from its sound one would never know which meaning to assign to a homophone, even such common ones as *their-there, two-too* or *peace-*

piece. Further, there are some pairs of words in English which, though spelled the same, are pronounced differently according to their meaning. Examples include:

sow	(female pig)	*vs*	*sow*	(some seeds)
tear	(to rip)	*vs*	*tear*	(shed when crying)
bass	(the singer)	*vs*	*bass*	(the fish)
minute	(sixty seconds)	*vs*	*minute*	(very small)

The point about such "heterophonic homographs" (!) is that the correct pronunciation can only be given to the word *after* the appropriate meaning has been specified.

We have spent rather a long time on phonic mediation theory in order to give the reader a feel for the way that psychological theories can be tested and improved by new evidence and arguments. Before leaving phonic mediation theory, it is perhaps worth commenting that it was in some respects a good theory. It was good because it was an explicit theory of word recognition; it was good because it stimulated a lot of research (and also some thought) about how we pass from print to meaning; and, last but not least, it was good because it was capable of being proved wrong by data and arguments. It is not always clear that the same can be said of some of the more complex and sophisticated accounts of reading which have replaced phonic mediation theory.

READING BY EYE

Because of the sort of arguments just presented it is by now almost universally accepted that when skilled readers recognize familiar words they do so "by eye" rather than (or, at least, as well as) "by ear." That is, readers recognize known words *visually*, as familiar letter strings. This amounts to the proposal that readers build up recognition units which recognize the written forms of familiar words. These are like the auditory word recognition units discussed earlier, but they identify letter codes rather than acoustic codes. So, as a new word becomes familiar through repeated encounters, a *visual word recognition unit* is created whose job it is to respond to, or be activated by, the newly learned word each time it is encountered on the printed page. Skilled readers must possess thousands of such units within their *visual word recognition systems.*

Once a visual word recognition unit is established that word need no longer be sounded out before being identified. Alphabetic regularity is not a concern when reading by eye because this method of reading exploits the word level of representation, having one recognition unit for each word (or possibly each morpheme—see Chapter 3). When words are recognized visually as wholes it is more important that they should be visually distinct than that they should be regular. The "direct" or "visual route" therefore benefits when homophones are spelled differently (like *sword* and *soared*, or *their* and *there*) and is probably inconvenienced by a word like *bank* which can mean either the side of a river or where you go for your money.

Recently a computer model of this visual mode of word recognition has been developed by Rumelhart and McClelland (1981; 1982; McClelland and Rumelhart, 1981) at the University of California in San Diego. Rumelhart and McClelland are not concerned to get a computer to recognize words by just any means; rather they have sought to incorporate in their program a theory of how *humans* recognize words. This means that the computer's performance on a variety of word recognition tasks is compared with the performance of human subjects. Where there is a discrepancy the model embodied in the program is modified until the performance of the computer falls into line with that of the humans.

The Rumelhart and McClelland model of direct visual word recognition

The Rumelhart and McClelland model (henceforth the R & M model) is complex, but we shall try to convey some indication here of how it works. A simple diagrammatic representation of the R & M model is shown in Figure 2.3.

The model is capable of identifying nearly 1200 four-letter words as long as they are written in a particular angular typeface where the letters are made up of straight lines without any curves. Basically the model consists of a visual analysis system and a visual word recognition system, but the analysis system is subdivided into a *feature level* and a *letter level*. The first thing to happen when a word is presented to the computer is that it tries to identify all the individual line features of which the letters are composed, and there is a different *feature detector* for each of the line features from which the letters are made up.

Suppose, for example, that the word TRIP is shown to the computer. The letter T contains a straight line across the top so the detector for the feature will become active. As it does so, its feature detector begins to activate all the letter detectors for letters with a straight line across the top (e.g., E, F, I, and T), but as well as activating detectors for letters with the feature it also begins to *inhibit* detectors for letters without a line across the top (e.g., H, L, N, Y). The interplay of activating and inhibiting connections is a characteristic of the R & M model. Now, T has a central vertical line so its letter level detector will also be activated by the appropriate feature detector. E and F do not contain *central* vertical lines so they will be inhibited. The computer's visual analysis system is capable

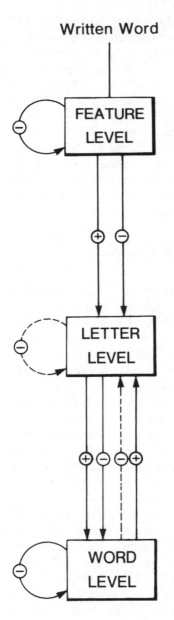

Written Word

FEATURE LEVEL
Features identified in individual letters. Feature detectors inhibit one another.

Feature detectors activate position-specific letter detectors containing their feature and inhibit all other letter detectors.

LETTER LEVEL
Individual letters identified. Letter detectors receive activatory and inhibitory inputs from feature detectors, and activatory inputs from word level units. Inhibition between letter detectors is permitted in the R & M model but not used in the simulations.

Letter detectors activate word recognition units containing their letter and inhibit all other units. Letter detectors are, in turn, activated by feedback from the word level. Word-to-letter level inhibition is permitted in the model but not always used in the simulations.

WORD LEVEL
Word recognition units respond to activatory and inhibitory inputs from the letter level and also mutually inhibit each other. The word recognized is the one whose activation level remains high while the others are suppressed.

Figure 2.3 A simplified representation of Rumelhart's and McClelland's model of direct visual word recognition (+ denotes an activatory connection, − denotes an inhibitory connection).

of identifying all four letters of a word simultaneously so, if all goes well, then a few milliseconds after the word TRIP has been displayed the feature detectors will have activated the appropriate set of four letter detectors and inhibited the others so the computer knows the word being shown contains the letters T, R, I, and P.

As the letter-level units for T, R, I, and P begin to be activated they in turn start to activate word level units. This is another important characteristic of the R & M model, that work at one level does not have to be completed before the next level can begin to be activated. The levels within the R & M model are described as being *in cascade*. This means that as soon as units at one level *begin* to become active they start to activate units at the next highest level, so that a lot can be happening up at the word level before even feature analysis is complete. This is not just cleverness—it has been found to be necessary in order to simulate human performance.

When TRIP is shown, the letter detector for initial T will start to activate the word level unit for TRIP, but it will also have activatory connections to the units for other words beginning with T such as TRAP, TAKE, and TIME. In fact, TRAP shares three letters in common with TRIP so will be quite highly activated by it. The set of other words which a presented word activates to some degree are called its *visual neighbors*. However, though the word-level unit for TRAP will be activated by the T, R, and P of TRIP, it will be inhibited by the I detector (whereas TRIP will be activated by it too). Letter-level units not only activate word units for words containing their letter but also inhibit or suppress activation in recognition units for words not containing their letter.

There is another source of inhibition we must contend with in the R & M model, and it concerns the fact that, as word-level units become activated, they seek to inhibit *each other*. That is, there are mutual inhibitory connections *between* word-level units. This is another device to ensure that when a word is read, although many word units may be momentarily activated, one and only one "wins" and remains active. That unit defines the word the computer reports as having been shown.

In one of the word recognition tasks the R & M model has been designed to simulate, subjects are shown very briefly a letter string which may or may not be a word. When the letter string disappears it is replaced by a "pattern mask" made up of jumbled letter fragments. After the pattern mask the subject is shown two letters and asked to indicate which of the two occurred in the initial letter string. For example, a subject might be shown TRIP followed by the mask, then R and S, and the subject's task is to indicate that the R but not the S was present in TRIP. In this task it has been shown that subjects perform best if the initial letter string is a real word like TRIP, less well if it is a "wordlike" nonword (or "pseudoword") like TREP, and worse still if it is a letter string like TPRI which could never be a word in English. What is of interest is that subjects are only being asked to say which of two *letters* was in the initial letter string, yet they do better if the letter string was a real word. In other words, they show a *word superiority effect* which seems to imply that skilled readers actually *see* letters more easily or more quickly when those letters form part of known words than when they do not.

To explain this word superiority effect Rumelhart and McClelland propose that, as well as the letter level influencing activity at the word level, the reverse can happen and the word level can affect the letter level. Word units have activating connections back to the letter recognizers responsible for identifying their component letters. So, when TRIP is presented, as soon as its word-level unit starts to be activated it in turn contributes activation to the letter recognizers for T, R, I, and P. These are now getting activation from downstream (the feature detectors) and upstream (the word unit for TRIP) and so the component letters are identified more quickly than if they had been presented as TPRI. In fact, to the extent that TRIP also momentarily activates its visual neighbors such as TRAP, TRIM, SHIP, etc., they too will contribute to the perceptual resolution of the letters in TRIP.

TREP may not be a word, but it has visual neighbors in TRIP, TRAP, etc., and these will contribute to the perception of its component letters. This is why letters in wordlike nonwords are better identified than letters in strings like TPRI. Wordlike does not necessarily mean pronounceable: SPCT has as many visual neighbors (SPIT, SPOT, SOOT, SECT, FACT, etc.) as SPET, and Rumelhart and McClelland showed that both human subjects and their computer perceive SPCT and similar unpronounceable letter strings as rapidly as they perceive pronounceable nonwords like SPET provided that the two types of letter string have the same numbers of visual neighbours. The reason TPRI is slow to be perceived is not because it is hard to pronounce but because it causes little activity up at the word level.

The different levels in the R & M model are distinct and separable, but constantly interacting, hence the R & M model is known as an *interactive activation model*. An interesting feature of such models is that they are also *compensatory models* because activity at one level can compensate for slowness or inefficiency at another level. We shall have cause to remember this aspect of interactive models when we look at the effects of context on word recognition (Chapter 5) and the development of word recognition skills in children (Chapter 7). The R & M model has many illustrious predecessors and some current competitors. One of its major successes has been the way it has shown that earlier models were not so much pie-in-the-sky, but incorporated concepts which were basically sound and which can be built into a working system. However, as Rumelhart and McClelland observe, although the interactive activation model is simple in essence, its actual behavior is complex and virtually impossible to predict without "running" it. Indeed, the model has proved to have unforeseen properties which have then been shown to be also true of people (an example being the importance of wordlikeness over pronounceability mentioned earlier).

Accessing meanings and pronunciations

The R & M model of direct (that is, not phonically mediated) visual word recognition ends with the identification of words. It does not (as yet) involve word meanings or word pronunciations. In humans, however, the very point of identifying a word you are reading is to allow you to understand the meaning it conveys and possibly to pronounce it as well. How are these meanings and pronunciations attained?

We assume that the next stage following activation of a *human* visual word recognition unit is the activation of a meaning. Linguists use the term *semantics* to refer to word meanings, so we could call the mental representation of a word's meaning a *semantic representation,* and we could call the system in which these representations are housed the *semantic system.* Although theories exist about what semantic representations might look like (Foss and Hakes, 1978; Kintsch, 1980) we shall not inquire too deeply into them because there is rapid change and little consensus. The notion of a semantic representation will still, however, be a useful one.

If the activation of a word recognition unit causes the word's meaning as encapsulated in its semantic representation to be activated, this still leaves us to explain how we can then pronounce the word. One possibility is that word names are accessed in the same way that we access pronunciations when naming objects or just talking spontaneously. Suppose you are asked to think of a domestic pet and name it. You may say "cat" or "Tiddles" or whatever. Presumably you have conjured up a particular memory and used that meaning to access the pronunciation. In order to get from semantic representations or codes to pronunciations we require a word production system. Semantic codes provide the input to that system, whose output is pronunciations. These are probably represented as strings of phonemes, that is the consonant and vowel sounds which are articulated when a word is spoken. Because the output of the word production system is strings of phonemes we shall call it the *phonemic word production system.* Although a word's phonemic form is retrieved as a unit, it must then be articulated "from left to right." Accordingly, we need a *phonemic buffer*; that is, a short-term store in which the phonemes of a word are held between being retrieved and being articulated. (It should not surprise us that in our attempts to understand visual word recognition we have been led into considering both speech perception and speech production. Reading is an artificial, culturally maintained skill which undoubtedly draws upon psychological systems and processes originally set up for handling spoken language.)

The model for visual word recognition which emerges from these considerations is shown in Figure 2.4. The feature level and letter level of the R & M model have been collapsed again into a single visual analysis system, and the word level is now referred to as the visual word recognition system. When a word is recognized its component letters are identified by the visual analysis system. Letter identification causes activity in the visual word recognition units until a combination of activation and inhibition causes one unit to remain active while the others are suppressed. That unit's sustained activity causes the appropriate semantic representation to be activated and the reader now knows the meaning of the word being read. The semantic representation may then activate the appropriate phonemic word production unit, releasing the phonemic form which is then available to be spoken if necessary. This sequence of operations has been described as if it were linear and sequential with processes at one level or stage being completed before processes at the next level or stage begin, but there is no reason why the whole sequence might not be "in cascade," with the beginning of activity at one level triggering other activities several stages further on down the line.

SUMMARY OF CHAPTER 2

Skilled readers possess a capacity for reading "by ear"; that is, for sounding out an unfamiliar written word to see if it sounds familiar in its spoken form. It is proposed that this "phonic route" to meaning involves (1) identifying the letters of a written word, (2) applying a knowledge of English letter-sound correspondences to create an internal acoustic form, and (3) identifying that acoustic code by means of auditory word recognition units, just as if the word had been heard. While all reading theories acknowledge reading "by ear" as an available route or strategy, phonic mediation theory proposed that is the *only* available route from print to meaning. Two lines of evidence were adduced against phonic mediation theory. These were:

1   that acquired phonological dyslexics are able to comprehend and pronounce familiar words despite having lost the capacity for letter-sound conversion; and

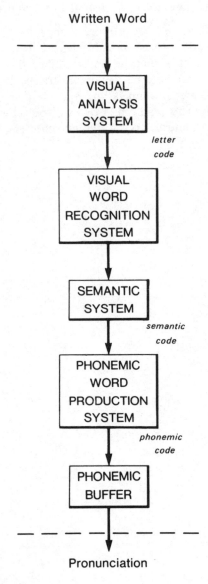

Figure 2.4 A model for the direct visual recognition, comprehension, and naming of familiar written words.

2   that phonic mediation theory cannot explain how we can assign the correct meanings to homophones like *boy* and *buoy*, or the correct pronunciations to homographs like *tear* (to cry) and *tear* (to shred).

It is necessary, therefore, to propose a capacity for reading "by eye" which allows letter codes to be directly identified by visual word recognition units. When such a unit becomes active, the word's meaning or semantic representation becomes available to the reader who can then access the appropriate pronunciation via phonemic word production units. This route used to read "by eye" will be referred to as the *direct route* to meaning in contrast to the *phonic route* employed when reading by ear.

3 Routes and Options in Word Comprehension and Naming

As mentioned in the previous chapter, the Rumelhart and McClelland model is just one of the latest in a long line of theories of word recognition (and a model is just the embodiment of a theory). One predecessor whose influence Rumelhart and McClelland explicitly acknowledge is the *logogen model* developed in a series of papers by John Morton at the Medical Research Council Applied Psychology Unit in Cambridge, England (e.g., Morton, 1964a; 1969; 1979a; 1979b; 1980; 1982). Morton uses the term *logogen* (from the Greek *logos* = word and *genus* = birth) for what we have called word recognition and word production units.

EVIDENCE FOR SEPARATE VISUAL AND AUDITORY WORD RECOGNITION SYSTEMS

In the logogen model each logogen (= visual word recognition unit) has a *threshold* which determines the amount of activation which must be present in that logogen before it will "fire" and provide access to the word's meaning and pronunciation. Each time a logogen fires its threshold is lowered slightly so that less stimulus information is needed to fire it next time. The Rumelhart and McClelland model has no concept of thresholds. Instead, word level units for common words have higher resting levels of activation than the units for uncommon words. The effect is the same for all intents and purposes, and makes the same important prediction which is that a single encounter with a relatively uncommon word should have a lasting and measureable influence on the future perceptibility of that word. This is known as *repetition priming*; it undoubtedly occurs, but it is subject to a very important limitation. To understand the importance of this limitation we must consider an early version of the logogen model in which individual logogens were responsible for the recognition and production of both the spoken and the written forms of a word (Morton, 1964a; 1969; 1979a). If each logogen recognized its own particular word whether that word was heard or read, then hearing an uncommon word should, by repetition priming, make that word subsequently easier to read, and vice versa. It is now known that this does not happen. Hearing a word primes later *auditory* recognition of the same word, and reading a word primes later *visual* recognition, but hearing does not prime later visual recognition and reading does not prime later auditory recognition (Morton, 1979b; Ellis, 1982a). In other words, repetition priming is *modality-specific,* and what *that* means is that if we are to retain something like Morton or Rumelhart and McClelland accounts of repetition priming then *we must have distinct auditory and visual word recognition units in distinct auditory and visual word recognition systems* (Morton, 1979b). These findings, then, justify what we have merely assumed so far, which is that the auditory word recognition system and the visual word recognition system are separate and separable.

THE ROLE OF MORPHEMES IN WORD RECOGNITION
AND PRODUCTION

Important as the Rumelhart and McClelland model is, it is presently restricted to identifying a vocabulary of single-morpheme, four-letter words. We saw in Chapter 1 that in English regular plural and past tense morphemes are spelled the same way despite variations in pronunciation (recall *ropes*, *robes*, *roses* and *flapped*, *soared*, *glided*). This would make sense if "bound morphemes" like -*s*, -*ed*, -*ing*, -*ly*, *un*-, or *dis*- were recognized separately from the "root morphemes" to which they are attached. There is some evidence that this may indeed happen.

If when we read *pains* and *pained* the bound morphemes -*s* and -*ed* are recognized separately from the root morpheme *pain*, then it follows that the same recognition unit probably recognizes the *pain* morpheme in *pain* itself and also in *pains* and *pained*. Thus, reading *pains* should prime later recognition of *pained* but should not prime later recognition of a visually similar word like *paint* since reading *pains* should cause no lasting change in the threshold or resting level of activation in the recognition unit for *paint*. This prediction was tested in an experiment by Murrell and Morton

(1974) who found that reading *pains* did indeed prime later recognition of *pained* but not of *paint*, just as reading *topped* and *bored* primed later recognition of *topping* and *boring* but not *topple* or *born*.

We should perhaps rechristen our recognition systems the "visual morpheme recognition system" and the "acoustic morpheme recognition system," but we shall stick to the old names to avoid confusion. Interestingly, the phonemic word production system used in speaking also appears to be morphemically organized. Garrett (1982) makes this point when discussing slips of the tongue such as the one made by the speaker who meant to say, "She slants her writing" but instead said, "She writes her slanting." In this error the *slant* morpheme from *slants* has exchanged places with the *write* morpheme of *writing* leaving the bound morphemes *-s* and *-ing* stranded. Such errors imply that morphemes have their own units in the phonemic word production system. Given that we can have no inborn mechanisms for processing written language, when a recognition system is established for reading it is probably set up using principles and processes derived from the recognition of speech. Having morphemic rather than word recognition and production units greatly reduces the number of units required, which is why computer systems for reading text often utilize this principle (e.g., Allen, 1980).

NAMING WORDS

In the previous chapter we rejected phonic mediation as a theory of how skilled readers recognize familiar words and replaced it with a model permitting direct visual access to meanings and phonemic forms. However, the phonic mediation model had certain desirable features which the direct visual access model has lost. In particular the phonic mediation theory could explain how we can comprehend unfamiliar letter strings of the *phoks* type. It is now time to consider again the relationship between the comprehension and the pronunciation of print, and how we might adapt the visual access model so as to re-introduce the better features of phonic mediation theory.

Addressed and assembled pronunciations

One way to pronounce a written word using the direct route is to go via the word's meaning. Here the word's meaning (its semantic representation) is used to retrieve the pronunciation *as a whole* from the phonemic word production system. The semantic representation or code may be said to *address* the appropriate word production unit, so we may talk of this mode of word naming as involving *addressed pronunciation*.

Although naming via meaning is one way of achieving an addressed pronunciation, recent neuropsychological research suggests it may not be the only way. Schwartz, Marin, and Saffran (1979) and Schwartz, Saffran, and Marin (1980) describe in detail a sixty-two-year-old woman (initials W. L. P.) who was suffering from a progressive presenile dementia, including a generalized loss of memory. At one stage in her illness W. L. P. was quite unable to match written animal names against their appropriate pictures. When presented with twenty low-frequency animal names such as *hyena*, *leopard*, and *llama*, together with some names of body parts and some colour names, she could only sort out seven of the twenty animal names as referring to animals at all. Nevertheless, she managed to read aloud eighteen of the twenty animal names, including the three mentioned above, and made only minor stress placement errors on the other two (*rhinoceros* read as "rhinoCERos" and *buzzard* as "buzZARD").

In general W. L. P. displayed a remarkable capacity to read words aloud despite showing very little evidence of understanding many of them, and despite being quite unable to use them in her own limited spontaneous speech. Nevertheless, until the final stages of her illness she could read aloud regular and irregular words with equal impunity and could also read nonwords aloud. W. L. P. was not reading real words by letter-sound conversion, but her meaning system was so impoverished as a consequence of her dementia that it is unlikely to have been able to sustain reading via meaning. The explanation favoured by Schwartz, Saffran, and Marin is that W. L. P. was reading words aloud with the aid of one-to-one connections between visual word recognition units and phonemic word production units.

The proposal that reading without meaning uses one-to-one connections between visual word recognition units and phonemic word production units is the best account currently available. However, some psychologists are reluctant to draw conclusions about normal processing solely on the basis of such case studies. It is obviously better if such a proposal could also explain some observations on normal people. Warren and Morton (1982) think it can. They draw attention to experiments by Potter and Faulconer (1975) which showed that it takes normal subjects longer to name a picture than to read a word. This cannot be because it takes longer to *identify* pictures than words since normal subjects took *less* time to judge whether a picture depicted an animate or inanimate object than to judge the equivalent word. Warren and Morton suggest that these results can be explained if objects are always named via their meaning whereas direct connections between visual word recognition units and phonemic word production units can by-pass that stage for naming written words. This proposal is still being debated (see Ratcliff and

Newcombe, 1982), but illustrates the kind of fruitful theoretical inter-action which can exist between neuropsychological and experimental cog-nitive research.

If we are prepared to accept this evidence for one-to-one connections, then our model of reading now has *two* methods of accessing addressed pronunciations, one via meaning and one via the connections between recognition and production units. We still lack, however, a device for assembling pronunciations to fit new words or nonwords.

Routes to "assembled" pronunciations

When a new and unfamiliar word is encountered in a passage (or an experiment) its pronunciation cannot be addressed, but must be assembled. (The terms "addressed" and "assembled" pronunciation are from Patterson, 1982.) How is this done? Suppose you are shown the nonword *nade* and asked to pronounce it. *Nade* will not fully activate any visual word recognition units for visually similar real word neighbours like *name*, *made*, and *fade*. By virtue of the one-to-one connections be-tween visual word recognition units and phonemic word production units the partial activation caused by *nade* should release the phonemic forms of those neighbours, and from those phonemic forms a candidate pronun-ciation for *nade* can be assembled.

The mode of assembling pronunciations just described exploits similarities between new and familiar words, and hence has been de-scribed as pronunciation *by analogy* (Glushko, 1979). For a nonword like *nade* the process is relatively straightforward, but a nonword such as *mave* presents greater difficulties. This is because *-ave* is pronounced one way in *gave*, *pave*, *wave*, etc. but a different way in the very frequent word *have*. That is, *-ave* affords rival and *inconsistent* analogies. If pronunciations for new words are assembled by analogy, then nonwords containing consistently pronounced letter strings should be named more rapidly than nonwords which contain inconsistently pronounced letter strings, since in the latter case some sort of decision must be made be-tween the rival analogies.

The analogy theory of pronunciations was formulated by Glushko (1979) who also tested its predictions. Glushko showed that nonwords which incorporate inconsistent letter-sound correspondences are indeed pronounced more slowly than consistent nonwords, just as analogy theory predicts. He also showed that consistent real words like *blade* are pro-nounced faster than other familiar words like *brave* which contain in-consistently pronounced letter strings. This implies that analogies may contribute to (and sometimes retard) even the naming of familiar words.

Further evidence favoring analogies over rules as means of letter-to-phoneme conversion has been provided by Kay and Marcel (1982). They showed that one can influence how an inconsistent nonword is read aloud be preceding it with real words containing one or other of the rival correspondences. For example, if *mave* is preceded by *wave* in a list of mixed words and nonwords, then *mave* will usually be read so as to rhyme with *wave*. If, however, *mave* is preceded by *have* then it will sometimes (though not always) be read so as to rhyme with *have*. This finding lends itself to an explanation in terms of analogy theory, where the particular analogy used to pronounce a new word can be influenced by recent experience of visually similar known words.

Now, analogy theory is fine when we are discussing the naming of short unfamiliar nonwords like *nade* and *mave*, or even long nonwords like *flambulance* and *flippopotamus* for which analogies are readily available. But what if the new word one is trying to pronounce is a name like *Glushko*, *Zbigniew Brzezinski*, or *Kishkemunasee*, or a Russian placename like *Atkyubinsk* or *Dnepropetrovsk*? While one may make use of, say, the *lush* in *Glushko*, or the *prop* in *Dnepropetrovsk*, much of the letter-sound conversion involved in pronouncing such words must operate down at the syllable or even the single-letter level.

The picture of assembled pronunciation which emerges from these considerations is one in which readers use the *largest available visual segment* when assembling pronunciations. If the new word is simply two familiar words joined together (e.g., *swallowtail* or *sparrowhawk*), then the new pronunciation will be *assembled* from two word pronunciations which are themselves *addressed*. Where words are not present, morphemes may be; for example, the pronunciation of *anti-* would probably be addressed as a unit then combined with an assembled phonemic form for *macassar* to create a pronunciation for *antimacassar* by someone not familiar with this term for a decorated cloth used to protect the back of a chair. Where no familiar words or morphemes are embedded in a new word, analogies with visual neighbors may still be used, as is implied by the results of Glushko (1979) and Kay and Marcel (1981) mentioned earlier. Finally, when necessary readers will resort to a syllable-by-syllable or even letter-by-letter process of assembly. Here the letter string will be scanned from left to right and broken down into pronounceable subunits. The phonemic equivalents of these letter groups will be assembled, then "blended" together into a pronunciation.

Comprehending an assembled pronunciation

A tenet of phonic mediation theory was that after a written word had been sounded out and converted into an acoustic code, that code was then identified by the auditory word recognition system just as if the word had been heard. Though we have rejected phonic mediation as an obligatory stage in reading, we may still wish to retain this account of the final comprehension of assembled pronunciations. Indeed an unpublished experiment by Peter Gipson at the Medical Research Council Applied Psychology Unit in Cambridge supports this proposal. Gipson showed that although reading conventionally spelled familiar words like *fox* or *yacht* does not prime later auditory word recognition of the spoken words "fox" and "yacht," reading phonically misspelled words like *phoks* or *yott* for meaning *does* improve later identification of the spoken words heard against a background of noise. This must be because reading for meaning on the phonic route involves activating auditory word recognition units in a way that reading for meaning on the direct, visual route does not.

We have argued that phonemic forms are assembled and held in some pre-articulatory form (in a short-term phonemic buffer store, equivalent to the *response buffer* in Morton's logogen model—see Ellis, 1979a). How is that phonemic form converted into an acoustic code capable of being identified by the auditory word recognition system? It could, of course, be pronounced aloud, but we do not need to do that to know that a *phoks* is an animal. When we "talk to ourselves" silently we seem to hear our own voices inside our heads. Perhaps that "inner speech" loop is what turns phonemic forms into acoustic codes to permit phonically mediated comprehension. We can easily show that this loop can participate in the comprehension of addressed as well as assembled pronunciations by demonstrating that readers can answer silently questions like *Does PAIR sound like a fruit?* or *Does SWORD sound like something an albatross might have done?*

THE FINAL MODEL

The final model of single word comprehension and naming which we are now ready to unveil owes much to the post-1979 version of Morton's logogen model (Morton, 1979b; 1980; 1982; also Seymour, 1979). The reason that Figure 3.1 does not wholeheartedly embrace the terminology of the logogen model is simply the wish to maintain a certain distance from current debates over rival models of word recognition. Our final model is complex, but then so is reading, and the model still does not include those processes which only come into operation when we are reading words combined into sentences, paragraphs, or books. The model emphasizes cognitive architecture—the layout and interconnections of the structures which make reading possible. Because it emphasizes *structure*, it must be complemented by an account of the *processes* which occur within each component; hopefully this chapter and the previous one have at least gone some way towards providing such an account. Though a structural model is of little or no use unless accompanied by descriptions of processes, it does help one keep in mind the total configuration of the whole and the connections between the parts. Model making is just a way of expressing a theory which could perfectly well be expressed in words, but a diagram somehow seems to capture the simultaneity of cognitive operations in a way verbal expression finds difficult. That said, nothing in this book stands or falls on whether or not the reader finds diagrams a natural means of communicating a theory.

We shall finish our consideration of word recognition by tracing the path taken through the model by two different sorts of letter strings.

1   Familiar written words. Most of the words a skilled reader encounters in print are words which have been met many times before and whose meaning and pronunciation are well known. Following visual analysis such words are identified by activation in their particular visual word recognition units. If the word being read contains more than one morpheme these are probably identified by separate recognition units. When a unit is activated it makes available the word's semantic representation. The appropriate phonemic form may be retrieved from the phonemic word production system either via the semantic representation or as a result of one-to-one connections between visual word recognition units and phonemic word production units. In reading aloud the phonemic form would then be articulated.

2.   Unfamiliar written words. An unfamiliar written word must first undergo visual analysis permitting its component letters to be identified. If the letter string is clearly not a possible word in English then processing need proceed no further, but under normal circumstances this will rarely happen. If the letter string is, say, a misprint in a newspaper it may still resemble the intended word closely enough to activate that word's recognition unit and one may "accept" it *as* the intended word. Because misprints can fire recognition units they often pass completely unnoticed—the so-called "proof reader's error."

On other occasions the unfamiliar letter string will clearly be one which has not been encountered before. One could take a more or less informed guess using the word's context as a clue to its possible identity, but skilled readers are probably more likely to resort to phonic mediation. Using the principle of the largest available visual segment they will exploit embedded words and morphemes, analogies, and correspondences in order to assemble a candidate pronunciation as a phonemic form. That phonemic form can then be converted into an acoustic code and submitted to the

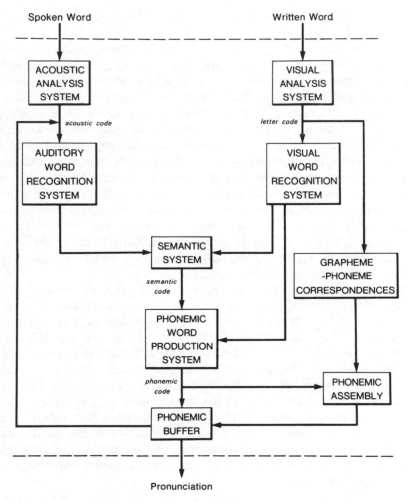

Figure 3.1 A model for both the direct and the phonically mediated recognition, comprehension, and naming of written words.

auditory word recognition system to see if the spoken form of the word "rings a bell." If the unfamiliar word is a reasonably regular one there is a chance that this route will succeed, particulary if several different candidate pronunciations are tried, and if the context in which the word occurs is used to prime likely auditory recognition units. Alas, however, if the word is an exceptionally irregular one even this strategy may fail. Of course the unfamiliar word may not even have been heard before, in which case no auditory word recognition unit will exist for it. Here all the reader can do is pronounce the candidate phonemic form aloud with a quizzical expression and intonation.

SUMMARY OF CHAPTER 3

If an uncommon word is read now it will be identified visually more easily or more rapidly in a subsequent test (the repetition priming effect). It is proposed that each encounter with a written word either lowers the threshold of the recognition unit for that word (as in the logogen model) or increases its resting level of activation (as in the Rumelhart and McClelland model). An important finding is that reading a word does not prime subsequent auditory recognition, and hearing a word does not prime subsequent visual recognition. This implies that the visual word recognition system is separate and distinct from the auditory word recognition system. A second important finding is that reading a word containing a particular root morpheme primes later visual recognition of other words containing the same root morpheme. This implies that recognition units may, if fact, be morpheme recognizers rather than (or as well as) word recognizers. Morphemes also appear to be separately represented in the phonemic word production system.

The phonemic forms (pronunciations) of familiar words are accessed as wholes ("addressed") either via the semantic representations or via one-to-one connections between visual word recognition units and phonemic word production units. Phonemic forms for unfamiliar words must be built up ("assembled"). Skilled readers appear to use the largest available visual segments to do this, and will convert letter strings to phonemic forms using words or morphemes embedded in the unfamiliar item, analogies with known words, or low-level syllable or grapheme-phoneme correspondences. Phonemic forms may be converted into acoustic codes (possibly using "inner speech") and tested to see if the word sounds familiar (phonically mediated comprehension). As a strategy phonic mediation is more likely to succeed if the new word is regularly spelled than if it is irregularly spelled.

4 The Acquired Dyslexias

The brain is the organ of the mind. It is also an organ of the body and, as such, is susceptible to injury and illness. The commonest cause of injury to the brain is a stroke; that is, a disruption of the blood supply to a part of the brain. We have known since the pioneering work of Paul Broca in the nineteenth century that language problems (including problems with reading) tend to occur after strokes affecting the left rather than the right half of the brain (in right-handed people). It is the left half, or hemisphere, of the brain which in most people is responsible for language abilities (Springer and Deutsch, 1981).

Disorders of speech comprehension or production which occur as a consequence of brain injury are known as *aphasias*. There are several recognized varities of aphasia depending upon the precise nature of the language problem (Kertesz, 1979). Aphasic patients will often experience reading difficulties which are part and parcel of their more general language impairments. Sometimes reading problems are the predominant or the only "symptom," or are not explicable solely by references to the spoken language aphasia. In both cases we would talk about the patient suffering from an *acquired dyslexia*.

Acquired dyslexia was studied in the late nineteenth century by neurologists such as Carl Wernicke, whom we have already met as an early exponent of phonic mediation theory. The past ten or fifteen years have witnessed a revival of interest in acquired dyslexia among cognitive psychologists. The approach they have adopted is to ask, "How might the component processes involved in *normal* reading be organized such that they would be prone to the particular patterns of breakdown which we can observe in cases of acquired dyslexia?'' Research has shown that there are several quite different types of acquired dyslexia just as there are different types of aphasia (see Coltheart, 1981; Patterson, 1981; and Newcombe and Marshall, 1982 for reviews). We have already encountered phonological dyslexia and "nonsemantic reading" in earlier chapters. In this chapter we shall not review every known type of acquired dyslexia in detail, but will concentrate on those with the clearest theoretical implications and those with which we will need to be acquainted when we come to look at possible similarities between developmental dyslexia and acquired dyslexia in Chapter 8.

VARIETIES OF ACQUIRED DYSLEXIA

Visually based dyslexias

Our survey of visual errors in Chapter 2 has shown that such errors can happen in more than one way. Case studies of acquired dyslexics have demonstrated that different patients will make different sorts of visual error, presumably because different parts of the visual route to word meanings are impaired in these patients. Allport (1977) observed how normal subjects will make "visual segmentation errors" when shown two or more words simultaneously but briefly (e.g., reporting "glade" when shown *glove* and *spade*). Shallice and Warrington (1977) describe an acquired dyslexic patient who made a great many such errors, even when given unlimited time to view the words. Shallice and Warrington call this syndrome *attentional dyslexia*, and it would appear to indicate impairment of the visual analysis system and/or its connections with the visual word recognition system.

Marshall and Newcombe (1973) and Newcombe and Marshall (1982) have described a different type of visual dyslexia. Their patient misread *cap* as "cob," *met* as "meat," and *rib* as "ride" which might be construed as an impairment of visual analysis were it not for the fact that the visually dyslexic patient would often correctly name all the letters in a word yet go on to misidentify it. These errors, or "paralexias" as dyslexic misreadings are sometimes called, might conceivably occur as a consequence of a lack of effective inhibition either from letter level to word level or within the word level itself. Either way the patient displays a marked tendency towards what Coltheart (1981) calls "approximate visual access"; that is, a tendency to accept as sufficient a less than perfect overlap between the word presented and the response given. Errors of approximate visual access occur in other forms of dyslexia, and also in normal readers, particularly young children (see Chapter 7).

Phonological dyslexia

We have already met phonological dyslexia in Chapter 2. In fact phonological dyslexia is hardly a form of dyslexia at all since the major deficit is in the reading of nonwords rather than real words. Certainly phonological dyslexia would not be detected if one were not on the lookout for it, which may explain why it has only been noticed and reported in recent years (Beauvois and Dérousné, 1979; Dérousné and Beauvois, 1979; Shallice and Warrington, 1980; Patterson, 1982; Funnell, 1983).

The characteristics of phonological dyslexia were discussed in Chapter 2. To repeat, these patients can read most familiar, real words with ease but are very poor at reading aloud even simple nonwords. Their symptoms suggest a substantial loss of the capacity for letter-to-phoneme conversion despite which they successfully read familiar words aloud. As mentioned in Chapter 2, this pattern of abilities and deficits is not compatible with phonic mediation theories of reading.

The phonological dyslexic patient A. M. reported by Patterson (1982) would sometimes misread "function words" like *with* or *then*, and made a fair number of so-called "derivational errors" such as misreading *applaud* as "applause," *recent* as "recently," and *fall* as "failure." However, neither of these problems was present in the phonological dyslexic reported in detail by Funnell (1983).

Reading without meaning

In Chapter 3 we met the Patient W. L. P., a sufferer from presenile dementia who was able to read words aloud without showing any hint of understanding the meaning of the words she read. W. L. P. could read irregular words with virtually the same facility as she read regular words, so she cannot have been using assembled pronunciations for these known words (though she could assemble pronunciations for nonwords). As a consequence Schwartz, Saffran, and Marin (1980) proposed that W. L. P. named words by virtue of one-to-one connections between visual word recognition units and phonemic word production units, and we have seen that once postulated these connections can explain hitherto puzzling aspects of normal performance.

Newcombe and Marshall (1982) use the term *direct dyslexia* to describe W. L. P.'s condition (because of the intact "direct" one-to-one connections). This is not a very happy term, one reason being that it incorporates a very recent theoretical explanation which may later be shown to be wrong, and another reason being that it is at least questionable whether W. L. P.'s reading should be described as "dyslexic" at all. Certain children who read aloud well despite poor comprehension are dubbed "*hyper*lexic," so W. L. P. might arguably be described as hyperlexic rather than dyslexic. We have chosen simply to call it "reading without meaning."

Surface dyslexia

Much of the modern interest in the acquired dyslexias stems from a seminal and classic paper by John Marshall and Freda Newcombe, "Patterns of paralexia: a psycholinguistic approach" (1973). In that paper Marshall and Newcombe described visual dyslexia along with two other varieties of acquired dyslexia, *surface dyslexia* and *deep dyslexia* (the latter syndrome is dealt with in the next section). In the case of surface dyslexia it is perhaps easiest to work from the diagnosis to the symptoms rather than the other way round.

Although surface dyslexia is a complex syndrome, one can go a considerable way toward explaining its characteristics if one accepts a model like the one shown in Figure 3.1 (p. 33) and if one then assumes:

1 That the brain injury suffered by the surface dyslexic has affected connections between the visual word recognition system and the semantic system.

2 That the surface dyslexic can still access the phonemic forms of many written words as wholes because of intact connections between visual word recognition units and phonemic word production units.

3 That on other occasions this route fails and the patient either assembles a phonemic form using analogies and/or grapheme-phoneme correspondences, or adopts a strategy of approximate visual access.

4 That however phonemic forms are derived they are comprehended phonically via the auditory word recognition system so that the patient comprehends the word in accordance with the way he or she pronounces it rather than its appearance.

To explain how this account comes about we must look at the reading of surface dyslexics and in particular at the sort of errors they make. We stated in point 3 above that surface dyslexics often appear not to recognize a word as a whole but resort to a strategy of "sounding out" in order to assemble a candidate pronunciation for the word. A patient reading at least some words this way is of course more likely to assemble the correct pronunciation when it is a regular word rather than an irregular word being tackled, and surface dyslexics are indeed more successful at reading aloud regular words than irregular words. For example, a patient reported by Shallice and Warrington (1980) read correctly thirty-six out of thirty-nine regular words, but only twenty-five out of thirty-nine irregular words.

The errors made by surface dyslexics also often look like unsuccessful attempts to assemble pronunciations. Sometimes the errors are nonwords, as when a patient reads *island* as "izland," *sugar* as "sudger," *recent* as "rikunt," or *broad* as "brode." Sometimes the errors are other real words as when a patient reads *disease* as "decease," *guest* as "just," *phase* as "face," or *grind* as "grinned." In either case the errors are typical "phonic approximations" to the target word; that is, pronunciations based on treating a word as if it were an alphabetically transparent one. Marshall and Newcombe (1973) sought to explain these regularizations as due to the unsuccessful application of grapheme-phoneme correspondence rules, but Marcel (1980) and Henderson (1982) have argued that they can be accounted for as well, if not better, in terms of the use of inappropriate analogies.

Leaving aside the question of *how* surface dyslexics assemble phonemic forms, there is no doubt that the meaning they ascribe to a word follows the pronunciation they give it, rather than following the word's appearance. In a celebrated example from Marshall and Newcombe (1973) a surface dyslexic patient misread *listen* as "liston," pronouncing the *t* which should be silent, and added, ". . . the famous boxer" (the reference being to Sonny Liston). On another occasion the same patient read *begin* as "beggin" and added, "that's collecting money." This is classic phonically mediated comprehension of assembled pronunciations of the *phoks-yott-howziz* type.

If we were to argue that all surface dyslexic reading is done by assembling pronunciations, then we would be hard pressed to explain how they still manage to read a fair proportion of irregular words aloud correctly. This is because the pronunciation of an irregular word must presumably be retrieved as whole rather than assembled piecemeal. Such addressing could in principle be done via semantic representations, but there is evidence to suggest that this is not what happens. A surface dyslexic reported by Newcombe and Marshall (1982) was asked to go through a list of words attempting to define each word after he read it. The list included the words *mown, some, bury*, and *four*. The patient pronounced each word correctly but defined *mown* as "to cry," *some* as "money," *bury* as "a hat, headgear," and *four* as "for you, for me, for anyone else." There are two important points to note here. The first is that *mown, some, bury*, and *four* are all homophones or near-homophones and that the patient gave a definition appropriate to the other member of the like-sounding pair (i.e., *moan, sum, beret*, and *for*). The second point is that the presented words are all irregular or inconsistent (compare *mown* with *down*, *some* with *home*, *bury* with *jury*, and *four* with *flour*). Their pronunciations must have been addressed as wholes even though they were then misinterpreted. The route taken by these words is presumably the same as that a normal reader will use if asked, "Does *sword* sound like something an albatross might have done?"

Now, the route to meaning via addressed whole-word pronunciations will only really come unstuck when the surface dyslexic is trying to pronounce and comprehend homophones or near-homophones. Presumably this route is the one which permits the *correct* naming and interpretation of many regular and irregular words. Why, then, do surface dyslexics sometimes have to assemble pronunciations with the attendant risk of error? One possibility is that some visual word recognition units have been lost or rendered inaccessible so that the words they would formerly have identified have to be handled some other way. An alternative possibility is that some links between visual word recognition units and phonemic word production units have been lost (or perhaps were never established). In this case, although a word may activate its recognition unit, the word's pronunciation can still only be attempted by assembly.

Even this does not complete our account of surface dyslexia because there are still other errors in which the patient looks to be adopting a strategy of approximate visual access like the visual dyslexics discussed earlier. Holmes (1973) describes four surface dyslexic patients who, in addition to making the sorts of errors we have already discussed, also made visual errors such as misreading *tough* as "thought," *precise* as "precious," *sing* as "sign," and *foreign* as "forgiven." Holmes comments that these errors are rapidly produced, in contrast to the other, laboriously assembled pronunciations. It would appear then that many surface dyslexics have three error-prone strategies for identifying written words. The first is to identify them on the basis of overlap between the letter code created by the word being attempted and the stored specifications of the visual word recognition units—a strategy prone to visual errors. The second strategy is to use direct connections between visual word recognition units and phonemic word production units to derive whole-word pronunciations which are then fed to the auditory word recognition system for identification—a strategy prone to homophone errors of the *some* = "money" type. The third and final strategy is to assemble a pronunciation piecemeal, treating the word as new and unfamiliar. This strategy has a greater chance of success with regular words, and so leads to the characteristically superior performance of surface dyslexics on regular over irregular words, and the equally characteristic "regularizations" of irregular words.

The main symptoms of surface dyslexia—problems with irregular words, problems with homophones, 'regularization' errors—should ring a bell. They are precisely the difficulties we said in Chapter 2 that any model of reading incorporating obligatory phonic mediation would have. This is, of course, *because* surface dyslexics are reading predominantly, if not exclusively, by phonic mediation. The difficulties experienced by surface dyslexics confirm our belief in the inadequacy of phonic mediation as a theory of normal, skilled word recognition.

We have dwelt at length on surface dyslexia. One reason is that it is the sort of syndrome which challenges and taxes models of normal functioning and stimulates development of those models. Another reason is that parallels have recently been drawn between acquired surface dyslexia and the reading of normal young children, and also between surface dyslexia and some cases of developmental dyslexia. We shall consider these parallels in Chapter 7 and Chapter 8 where we shall also discuss the possible existence of developmental counterparts of the next variety of acquired reading disorder, deep dyslexia.

Deep dyslexia

Imagine yourself seated at a table in a hospital room. Opposite you is a patient who has suffered a stroke but who is alert and interested. You have brought along a pack of plain cards each of which has a single word written on it. You hold up a card bearing the word *ape*. "Can you read this word aloud for me?" you ask. "Certainly." replies the patient, "that's 'monkey.'" The next card you hold up bears the word *soul*, which the patient reads as "soup." He then goes on to read *baby* correctly, *lovely* as "loving," *his* as "in," *forest* as "trees," *window* correctly, *boap* as "don't know," *chance* as "don't know," *sympathy* as "orchestra," *signal* as "single," *quite* as "perhaps," *belief* as "pray," *was* as "one of those little words—don't know," *when* as "chick," and *building* as "builder."

If this did indeed happen to you, then you would know you were sitting opposite a *deep dyslexic*. The reading attempts presented above—all of them genuine—illustrate most of the cardinal "symptoms" of deep dyslexia. Deep dyslexics find words like *baby*, *church*, or *table*, which have concrete, imageable referents, easier to read than abstract words like *belief*, *truth*, or *justice*. Like the phonological dyslexics, deep dyslexics also find new or nonwords virtually impossible to read aloud.

Deep dyslexics make several different types of reading error. First and most striking are the semantic errors such as misreading *ape* as "monkey," *forest* as "trees," or *belief* as "pray." Secondly there are visual errors reminiscent of those made by visual dyslexics and surface dyslexics (e.g., reading *soul* as "soup" or *signal* as "single"). A third type of error appears to be a combination of a visual error followed by a semantic error (e.g., *sympathy* read as "orchestra" via *symphony*, and *when* read as "chick" via *hen*). Fourthly, there are the derivational errors (e.g., *lovely* read as "loving" and *builder* read as "building"). Fifth and last are the function word substitutions (e.g., reading *his* as "in" or *quite* as "perhaps"). Grammatical "function words" like these create difficulties for deep dyslexics despite the fact that they are some of the commonest words in the language, but the errors made usually involve substituting another function word. (Derivational errors and function word substitutions were also made by the phonological dyslexic patient, A. M.) Table 4.1 shows a larger sample of deep dyslexic reading errors.

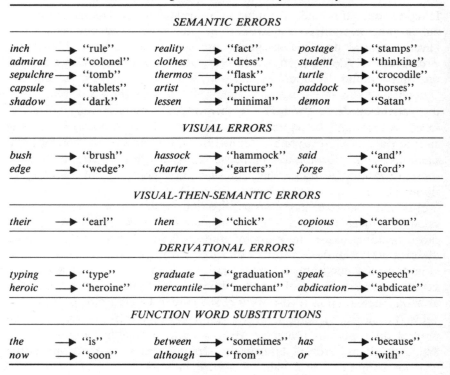

TABLE 4.1

Examples of deep dyslexic reading errors (taken from patients P.W. and D.E. reported by Karalyn Patterson in Appendix 2 of Coltheart, Patterson, and Marshall, 1980). The word in italics to the left of the arrow is the word shown to the patient and the word in inverted commas to the right of the arrow is the patient's response.

SEMANTIC ERRORS

inch → "rule"		*reality* → "fact"		*postage* → "stamps"	
admiral → "colonel"		*clothes* → "dress"		*student* → "thinking"	
sepulchre → "tomb"		*thermos* → "flask"		*turtle* → "crocodile"	
capsule → "tablets"		*artist* → "picture"		*paddock* → "horses"	
shadow → "dark"		*lessen* → "minimal"		*demon* → "Satan"	

VISUAL ERRORS

bush → "brush"		*hassock* → "hammock"		*said* → "and"	
edge → "wedge"		*charter* → "garters"		*forge* → "ford"	

VISUAL-THEN-SEMANTIC ERRORS

their → "earl"		*then* → "chick"		*copious* → "carbon"	

DERIVATIONAL ERRORS

typing → "type"		*graduate* → "graduation"		*speak* → "speech"	
heroic → "heroine"		*mercantile* → "merchant"		*abdication* → "abdicate"	

FUNCTION WORD SUBSTITUTIONS

the → "is"		*between* → "sometimes"		*has* → "because"	
now → "soon"		*although* → "from"		*or* → "with"	

Although patients with symptoms like those of deep dyslexia have been reported from time to time over the years (Marshall and Newcombe, 1980a), the first full descriptions were provided by Marshall and Newcombe (1966) and again in the same 1973 paper in which visual dyslexia and surface dyslexia were reported. Marshall and Newcombe adopted the same approach to explaining deep dyslexia as they took to explaining visual and surface dyslexia; that is, in terms of impairment to components of a model of normal reading. This approach has been developed further in papers by Newcombe and Marshall (1980), Morton and Patterson (1980), and Shallice and Warrington (1980).

For a start, their almost complete inability to read nonwords aloud suggests that deep dyslexics have lost the capacity for grapheme-phoneme conversion. Marshall and Newcombe have suggested that this loss alone may be sufficient to cause semantic errors to occur. They argue that reading via meaning may be inherently prone to substituting incorrect pronunciations which are similar in meaning to the target word and that, in normal readers, semantic errors are prevented from happening by the simultaneous activity of the grapheme-phoneme route. Thus, they argue, a normal reader will not read *forest* as "trees" because he or she knows that the correct pronunciation must start with an "f" sound. In reply to this one might note that phonological dyslexics have also lost the capacity for grapheme-phoneme conversion yet do not make semantic errors (though one could conceivably respond in turn by suggesting that phonological dyslexics retain error-checking one-to-one connections between recognition and production units which may also be lost in deep dyslexics).

If Marshall and Newcombe are wrong then the semantic systems of deep dyslexics may be impaired in some way. Indeed this proposal may be necessary to explain why abstract words are found to be so difficult. One can show that deep dyslexics still recognize abstract words *as words* by demonstrating that if a patient is given a set of cards on which are written either abstract words or nonwords then he may able to sort them into words and nonwords fairly accurately (Patterson, 1979), so the problem must be a more central one. It is possible that the difficulty with function words arises because they too are relatively abstract, though Morton and Patterson (1980) prefer to link the problem with function words with the occurrence of derivational errors, arguing that certain grammatical processes are impaired.

What is clear from the above is that an explanation of deep dyslexia in terms of damage to the normal reading process will have to postulate several different impairments. Also, we need to know more about the language skills of deep dyslexics outside of reading. For example, one patient reported by Friedman and Pearlman (1983) made semantic errors when naming objects as well as when naming words, supporting Shallice's and Warrington's (1980) contention that word retrieval problems may be the cause of semantic errors in at least some deep dyslexics.

However, the appropriateness of such an account of deep dyslexia has been challenged by Coltheart (1980b; 1983) who argues that in deep dyslexia we are not seeing the effects of partial impairment to the normal, left hemisphere reading processes. Instead Coltheart argues that in deep dyslexics the left hemisphere reading processes have been completely destroyed and the remaining word identification abilities are largely those of the right hemisphere, abilities which are dormant or supplementary in the intact adult (see also Saffran, Bogyo, Schwartz, and Marin, 1980). Although the left hemisphere is the one normally considered dominant for language, the right hemisphere of the brain appears to have certain, limited word recognition abilities. In essence Coltheart argues that the limitations of deep dyslexic word recognition are the limitations of the normal right hemisphere but that the deep dyslexic's speech comes from the left hemisphere. We shall not seek to arbitrate between Coltheart's "right hemisphere hypothesis" of deep dyslexia and the alternative view that it arises from partial impairment of the normal, dominant reading system, though it is worth noting that if Coltheart is right, studying deep dyslexia may not teach us much about normal reading processes (but see Shallice and Warrington, 1980, and Patterson and Kay, 1983, for objections to the right hemisphere hypothesis).

GENERAL ISSUES

There are a number of general points which are perhaps worth making at this juncture. First, when developing our theory of skilled word recognition in Chapters 2 and 3 we assumed that the right way to explain reading is through the combined activity of many separate but interacting components. These components (e.g., the visual analysis system, the auditory word recognition system, the processes of phonemic assembly, etc.) may be termed *modules*, and it has been argued—for example, by Marr (1976) and Allport (1980)—that all of our cognitive abilities should be explained in terms of such modules. The acquired dyslexias reinforce our belief in the correctness of this approach because they lend themselves so readily to explanations of the "modules *a*, *b*, and *c* are impaired while *x*, *y*, and *z* are intact" kind. Indeed it is hard to see how many different varieties of acquired dyslexia could occur if the underlying psychological processes did not have a fundamentally modular organization. Further, studying the acquired dyslexias may provide clues as to just what the separate modules are and how they interconnect. This is one reason why cognitive psychologists are becoming so interested in disorders of cognitive skills (Ellis,1982b).

Another important point to note is that although several distinctly different types of acquired dyslexia have been described, this does *not* mean that every patient who experiences reading problems after brain injury will fall neatly into one or other of the recognized categories. Patients will often show *mixed* symptoms; for example, visual difficulties *and* problems with letter-to-phoneme conversion combined perhaps with problems reading less common words by the direct route. The cases described in literature tend to be the small proportion of comparatively "pure" cases. Even so, there are individual differences between patients grouped together as "phonological dyslexics" or "surface dyslexics." Nevertheless, the simple fact that pure cases exist and have been documented establishes the existence of *varieties* of acquired dyslexia. The separate fact that many patients show hybrid symptoms does nothing to invalidate the claim that pure strains exist. We shall have reason to remember this point when we come to consider the possibility that varieties of developmental dyslexia may also exist.

SUMMARY OF CHAPTER 4

Injury to the language-dominant (usually left) hemisphere of the brain can result in a wide variety of different disorders of reading known as the acquired dyslexias. "Pure forms" of the different syndromes only occur in a minority of patients; the typical left-hemisphere injured patient will probably have multiple reading problems combined with other, more general language difficulties. That said, it is the rarer, pure cases which are most informative to the cognitive psychologist.

Because the different varieties of acquired dyslexia can be rather hard to remember, and because we shall be constantly referring back to them in later chapters, the types covered in this book are drawn together in Table 4.2. (For completeness the syndrome of letter-by-letter reading is included in Table 4.2 although it is not dealt with until Chapter 6.) It must be emphasized that Table 4.2 does not exhaust the recorded varieties of acquired dyslexia—several others have already been described and there are doubtless others to come.

The sheer existence of so many forms of acquired dyslexia with such varied characteristics provides strong support for the notion that the cognitive abilities of normal people are made possible by the concerted and orchestrated activity of many cognitive subcomponents or modules which nevertheless remain separate and dissociable.

TABLE 4.2
Varieties of acquired dyslexia (see Coltheart, 1981; Patterson, 1981; and Newcombe and
Marshall, 1982, for reviews)

1. Attentional dyslexia (alias literal dyslexia).
   Patient makes frequent visual segmentation errors when shown groups of words.
   Difficulty naming letters in strings but not letters in isolation.

   Main reference: Shallice and Warrington (1977).

2. Letter-by-letter reading (alias word-form dyslexia).
   Patient appears to name each letter of a word either aloud or subvocally before
   identifying the word, therefore reading time increases with the number of letters in
   the word. According to Warrington and Shallice (1980) reading is mediated via the
   patient's intact *spelling* system.

   Main references: Warrington and Shallice (1980); Patterson and Kay (1983).

3. Visual dyslexia.
   Patient makes frequent visually based errors in word recognition despite sometimes
   being able to name all the component letters of the target word. Deficit possibly due
   to "slippage" within the visual word recognition system.

   Main references: Marshall and Newcombe (1973); Newcombe and Marshall (1982).

4. Phonological dyslexia
   Patient is able to read many familiar words aloud with understanding, though may
   have some problems with function words and inflected words. No effects of regularity, imageability, or length. Virtually unable to read unfamiliar words or nonwords
   aloud suggesting impairment of grapheme-phoneme conversion and/or phonemic
   assembly.

   Main references: Beauvois and Dérousné (1979); Shallice and Warrington (1980);
   Patterson (1982).

5. Non-semantic reading (alias direct dyslexia).
   Occurs in some patients having "presenile dementia." Intact word naming (and
   apparently nonword naming) despite a lack of any indication that the patient under-
   stands the words being read. Arguably reading aloud is sustained by intact connections between visual word recognition units and phonemic word productions units
   despite disintegration of the semantic system.

   Main references: Schwartz, Marin, and Saffran (1979); Schwartz, Saffran, and
   Marin (1980); Shallice, Warrington, and McCarthy (1983).

6. Surface dyslexia (alias semantic dyslexia).
   Patient appears to read by phonic mediation. Some whole-word reading retained,
   but patient may misinterpret homophones showing that final access to the semantic
   system is via the auditory word recognition system. For many words the patient
   attempts to assemble a pronunciation with a consequent liability to "phonic" errors;
   other errors appear to be visual approximation similar to the errors of visual
   dyslexics. Regular words are read more successfully than irregular words. Principal
   deficits appear to be disconnection of visual word recognition system from the
   semantic system together with unavailability either of some visual word recognition
   units or some connections between those units and the corresponding phonemic
   word production units.

   Main references: Marshall and Newcombe (1973); Marcel (1980); Shallice and
   Warrington (1980); Henderson (1982).

7. Deep dyslexia (alias phonemic dyslexia).

   A complex syndrome whose central, defining symptom is the occurrence of semantic errors in single-word reading. Other symptoms include visual, visual-then-semantic and derivational errors, difficulty reading abstract words and function words, and an almost total inability to read nonwords. Several components of the reading system have been lost (e.g., Morton and Patterson, 1980), and Coltheart has argued that the remaining reading capacities are largely those of the right hemisphere.

   Main references: Marshall and Newcombe (1973); Coltheart, Patterson, and Marshall (1980).

5 Words in Combinations

So far in this book we have largely limited discussion to the reading of individual words by skilled readers, and to those acquired dyslexias whose characteristics can be adequately captured by models of single word reading. It is now time to acknowledge that most of the words we read in everyday life occur in the context of a text, such as a newspaper or book. In this chapter we shall focus on the psychological processes which reveal themselves when words are read in combinations.

We shall begin by examining the nature of eye movements in reading and the amount of information that can be taken in at a single glance. We shall then discuss the intricacies of sentence and text comprehension, and the argument that understanding a text involves reducing it to a set of underlying "propositions." The issue of whether we use the context preceding a word to assist in recognizing it will then be considered, followed by discussion of the nature of reading aloud, and, finally, the role of silent, inner speech in reading. These are all aspects of the processing of words in combinations.

EYE MOVEMENTS IN READING

As you sit engrossed in a good book your eyes seem to move smoothly and evenly along each line of print. This sensation of smooth eye movement is actually quite illusory because what your eyes really do is progress along the line in a sequence of rapid jerks with pauses between each jerk. The true nature of these reading eye movements was first observed in the nineteenth century by a French eye doctor called Javal, and these movements have been the object of intensive study ever since (see Rayner, 1978; 1983; and Mitchell, 1982, for reviews).

The rapid jerks by which the eyes move along a line are known as *saccades*. An average saccade lasts a mere twenty to fifty milliseconds (between a fiftieth and a twentieth of a second). The pauses between saccades are called *fixations*. These vary considerably in duration, but for the normal reader a typical fixation will last 200 or 250 milliseconds (between a fifth and a quarter of a second). Thus, despite the illusion of continuous movement, our eyes are actually *still* for about ninety percent of the time when we read.

The effective visual field

The eyes take in information only when they are still. When reading a novel or similar material an average reader will make five or six fixations along a typical line of print. This gives a clue as to the size of the "effective visual field"—that is, the size of the area around the fixation point from which we can absorb usable information about the words and letters on the page we are reading. Further down this page (don't look now!) is a line of print on its own. In the middle of that line is an *x*. In a moment (not yet) move your eyes directly to the *x*. The question is, how many letters or words can you see clearly enough to recognize? Ready . . . Now. If you held your eyes fixedly on the *x*, then to the right of it you probably saw the word *chair* clearly, together with the first few letters of *tomorrow* beyond. You will not have seen *that* well enough to recognize it, though you may have picked up its approximate shape

yacht bottle neighbor x chair tomorrow that

and length. To the left of the *x* you could probably only make out the *-or* of *neighbor* with some rough impression of the number of letters preceding the *-or*. Again, if you carried out the demonstration properly you would not have identified *yacht* or *bottle*.

Experiments using computer-controlled text displays have confirmed the veracity of these introspective observations. The "effective visual field" or "perceptual span" in reading is a mere ten or twelve letters or spaces (normally around two words). One picks up more information to the right of the fixation point than to the left (Rayner, Well, and Pollatsek, 1980). Perhaps because of this, the eyes usually alight about one-third of the way along a fixated word rather than in the middle or at the right end. Short, predictable words like *a* or *the* are often passed over in a saccade (O'Regan, 1979).

Reading rate and comprehension

With fixations of around 200–250 milliseconds and saccades of 20–50 milliseconds, the skilled reader should be able to achieve a comfortable reading rate of 1,000 words per minute or more. While this can sometimes be managed, the normal reading rate is a mere 200 to 400 words per minute. There are basically two reasons for this. First, some ten to twenty percent of reading eye movements are *regressions*; that is, backward movements in a right-to-left direction. Second, although the typical fixation is around a quarter of a second, some are much longer than this. Fixations tend to be longer on unfamiliar words which may indicate a switch from direct, visual recognition to phonically mediated recognition. Fixations also tend to be longer in grammatically complex sentences, and at the end of sentences in general, reflecting the ongoing grammatical and semantic processing of what is being read. Finally, as readers move from "easy" to "difficult" passages fixations tend to be longer, and the number of backward regressions increases.

The point is quite simply that the eyes can only progress as fast as the brain can absorb and comprehend what is being read. We can infer something about these processes of sentence and text comprehension by drawing on insights gained from several sources, most especially cognitive psychologists studying text comprehension and recall, and computer scientists attempting to program computers to answer questions based on passages of text.

COMPREHENDING WORDS IN COMBINATIONS

The first and most basic insight is that understanding the meaning of a passage involves much more than glueing together the meanings of the individual words it contains. For example, one must take note of the order of the words in a sentence. *The cat chased the rat* means something quite different from *The rat chased the cat*, yet the two sentences contain exactly the same words. Similarly, *Man bites dog* is news in a way that *Dog bites man* isn't. In these sentences, differences in meaning or function are signalled by differences in word order, and in English word order is determined by the role each word plays in its sentence. The examples just given depend upon the fact that the performer of an action normally becomes the grammatical subject of a sentence and is placed before the verb which expresses the action. The recipient of the action—in our cases the creature being chased or bitten—normally becomes the object of the sentence and is placed after the verb.

The rules of sentence structure are part of what is called the *syntax* of a language. Interestingly, there exists a group of brain-injured patients who have lost the capacity to utilize syntax or sentence structure in their comprehension. Shown a sentence like *The cat chased the rat*, these patients, known as *Broca's aphasics*, understand the meaning of each separate word, and so know that the sentence is about a cat and a rat, and that one chased the other, but because they cannot utilize word order they cannot say which animal is chasing which (see Saffran, 1982).

Now, Broca's aphasics experience the same language comprehension difficulties whether they are reading or listening to speech. This suggests that the same mechanisms for analyzing sentence structure are used in both reading *and* listening, so that most of the processes under discussion in this chapter are probably not specific to reading but are strategies for language comprehension in general. A further point is that while Broca's aphasics may have severe problems with *The cat chased the rat*, they can more easily understand *The cat chased the ball*, because a knowledge of the meanings of *cat*, *ball*, and *chased* is sufficient alone to allow that sentence to be understood (unless we are in the realm of fairy stories).

Sentence comprehension is an ongoing operation which uses both sentence structure and word meanings to formulate hypotheses about the meanings of the whole sentences. We certainly do not wait until a sentence has finished before analyzing and interpreting it. If this needs any illustration, then we can cite the case of so-called "garden path sentences" whose endings violate expectations built up at the beginning. An example from Foss and Hakes (1978) is the sentence, *The shooting of the prince shocked his wife since she thought that he was an excellent marksman*. We begin by assuming that the prince has been shot and that this shocked his wife, but the later portion of the sentence forces us to re-interpret the earlier part to mean that the wife was shocked because the prince was shooting badly.

Just as a later portion of a sentence may force us to re-interpret an earlier portion, so a later sentence may force us to re-interpret an earlier one. Sanford and Garrod (1981) illustrate this nicely. If you read *Jill came bouncing down the stairs. Harry rushed over to kiss her*, then you assign a particular meaning or image to the first sentence. If you then read *Jill came bouncing down the stairs. Harry rushed to fetch a doctor*, you probably begin by assigning the same meaning to *Jill came bouncing down the stairs*, but you have to revise that interpretation and assume a less happy meaning of *bouncing* when Harry rushes off.

A point the computer scientists were forced to acknowledge early on in their endeavors to program computers to "understand" stories is that even a grasp of word meanings and a knowledge of sentence structure are not sufficient to ensure the successful analysis of sentences. Take for instance the sentence *The city council refused the protestors a parade permit because they feared violence.* To whom does the word *they* refer? If you have arrived at a decision, try the sentence *The city council refused the protestors a parade permit because they advocated violence.* To whom does the word *they* now refer? Most people will say that *they* refers to the city council in the first sentence but to the protestors in the second sentence. Nothing in the sentence structure signals the change of referent of the word *they*; that change comes about because we know that in at least some parts of the world in which we live city councils are more likely to fear violence than to advocate it, and we can imagine scenarios in which a group of protestors seeking a parade permit might advocate violence. Winograd (1972), from whom this example is adapted, notes that if we want to program a computer to be able to correctly interpret sentences like these we would need to equip it not only with the rules of English syntax, but with all of the knowledge of the world that human listeners can bring to bear on sentence comprehension. For this reason work on computer story comprehension has concentrated on limited and well-regulated contexts such as goings-on in a restaurant where the computer *can* reasonably be equipped with much of the necessary general knowledge.

The products of comprehension

What happens when a sentence, or for that matter a story or a book, is comprehended? What are the *products* of comprehension? Recent summaries of research on sentence and story comprehension can be found in Bransford (1979), Danks and Glucksberg (1980), Sanford and Garrod (1981), and Mitchell (1982). If readers are presented with a story and then asked to recall it some time later they will often remember what we might call the *gist* of the story rather than its specific wording. Of course, one *can* memorize exact wording if that is important, but the more natural operation is probably the extraction and storage of gist. A similar conclusion is arrived at if you later present your readers with a set of sentences and ask them to indicate which were in the original story. They will often claim to recognize a sentence which preserves the gist of a sentence from the story but little of its wording. They will also claim to recognize new sentences containing information which was not present in the story but could reasonably be inferred from information which *was* provided.

So we remember a mixture of the original sentence or text information plus the information we add from our inferences. In what form is the information represented? A popular suggestion is that we boil the meaning of what we read down into a set of *abstract propositions* (see Mitchell, 1982). A proposition is a statement about a person or thing (e.g., *The dog is fat*), or about the relationship between two entities (e.g., *The dog chased the cat*). This means that, for example, the sentence *The fat dog chased the agile cat* contains three propositions:

1 The dog is fat.
2 The dog chased the cat.
3 The cat is agile.

These three propositions may be stored separately in memory, not as sentences in words, but as abstract representations which would, for example, be the same for the equivalent French or Spanish sentences. In remembering what we have read we recast these propositions into language, usually in our own words.

THE ROLE OF PRIOR CONTEXT IN WORD RECOGNITION

As we read we are actively building up a representation of the meaning encoded in the text in front of us by its writer. A question which has attracted considerable attention from cognitive psychologists is, "Do readers use the structure or meaning of the words they have just read to assist in identifying the word they are currently fixating?" Had this book been written two or three years ago, the answer given would almost certainly have been, "Yes, they do." That conclusion would have been based mainly on two lines of evidence. The first comes from experiments such as the one reported by Tulving and Gold (1963).

A word can be shown so briefly to a subject that he or she is unable to identify it. The exposure duration can then be gradually increased until the word is successfully identified. The particular exposure duration necessary for correct recognition is known as the word's *visual duration threshold*. Tulving and Gold measured the visual duration threshold of words presented either in isolation or after one, two, four or eight words of preceding context. The context words were either appropriate or inappropriate to the test word. So, in the eight-word appropriate context condition, subjects read a context such as *The skiers were buried alive by the sudden* and were then shown a target word such as *avalanche* very briefly. If the exposure was too brief and *avalanche* was not identified, the context was repeated and the target word was given a longer exposure. This continued until the target word was correctly recognized and its threshold was noted.

Tulving and Gold found that relevant context lowered visual duration thresholds; that is, it made the target words easier to identify. Increasing the amount of relevant context from one to eight words increased the size of the facilitation observed. Irrelevant context (e.g., *Medieval knights in battle were noted for their . . . avalanche*) actually made target words harder to identify than when they were presented in isolation with no preceding context—an inhibition effect. Similar results were reported by Morton (1964b).

The second line of evidence which has often been used to support the idea of contextual priming in reading originated in an experiment by Meyer and Schvaneveldt (1971). Subjects in this experiment had to decide whether presented letter strings were real words or not. Meyer and Schvaneveldt found that a letter string like *nurse* was accepted as a word more rapidly if it followed a related word like *doctor* than if it followed an unrelated word. This seemed to many to illustrate in simplified form the sort of contextual priming thought to occur in normal reading.

These are the lines of evidence which would probably have been used a few years ago to support the idea of contextual priming. However, a number of authors have recently argued cogently, and with evidence, against this idea (see Forster, 1981; Stanovich, 1981; Henderson, 1982; Mitchell, 1982). First, the Tulving and Gold procedure is somewhat remote from normal reading. The fact that the context is repeatedly presented for progressively longer intervals may encourage subjects to guess at the target word using the context and such letters from the target word as they think they may have perceived accurately. That is, reading *The skiers were buried alive by the sudden*, then seeing fleetingly a longish word beginning *av-* and ending *-he* may be enough to encourage many normal subjects to respond "avalanche." Such situations are not characteristic of normal, skilled reading.

Indeed, sentences with highly predictable final words are not commonly found in everyday texts. A typical incomplete sentence can be continued with many different words. As Forster (1981) observes, to use prior context one must be continuously enumerating and updating a set of contextually likely words and be priming their visual word recognition units. This would require a lot of computational work. Why should a skilled reader bother to go to all this effort for the sake of a few milliseconds saving in the recognition time of words, which is anyway a rapid and efficient process even for words in isolation. Similarly, few natural sentences contain closely associated pairs of words like *doctor-nurse*, an observation which must limit the extent to which the semantic priming demonstrated by Meyer and Schvaneveldt (1971) can be extrapolated to natural reading.

A situation where context *is* known to play an important role is speech perception (see Marslen-Wilson, 1980; Morton, 1979a). Speech differs from print in at least one important respect. Normal print constitutes a clear and clean stimulus, but the typical speech signal is a much more impoverished creature. Spoken words which are perceptible enough in context may be very hard to identify when extracted and played in isolation (Lieberman, 1963). When the incoming stimulus information is degraded, as it usually is in speech perception, then it may be worthwhile for an interactive system to utilize context predictively to aid ongoing word recognition. A skilled reader dealing with clear print is not in this situation and so is probably content to let the stimulus information drive recognition. Less skilled readers may, however, be in a position more akin to speech perception if their visual analysis or their input activation of visual word recognition units is slow or inefficient. The evidence on this point is inconsistent, and it is hard to be sure that poor (or young) readers do not rely more on phonic mediation, which may itself be capable of contexually priming, but Perfetti and Roth (1981) and Stanovich (1981) argue that less proficient readers make more use of context than do skilled readers.

One currently popular view is, therefore, that skilled readers do not use context predictively to anticipate likely continuations or prime recognition units. At least they do not do this when reading clear, everyday print such as is found in newspapers and books. They may conceivably use context when reading untidy handwriting which approximates to speech as a stimulus, but this speculation is as yet untested. Less skilled readers may utilize context predictively, but even this possibility is disputed (Mitchell, 1982).

ROUTES TO READING ALOUD

All the comprehension processes we have discussed so far in this chapter will occur whether one is reading silently or aloud. In this section we shall consider how pronunciations are derived when text is being read aloud, and in the next section we shall discuss the role of sound in silent reading.

From evidence already enumerated at length we can be confident that skilled readers do not access meanings via sound. Figure 3.1 (p. 33) still affords two routes to pronunciations that could be used to read aloud. The first is via word meanings, and the second is the direct connections between visual word recognition units and phonemic word production units for which we presented evidence in Chapter 3. The fact that when reading aloud we imbue sentences with appropriate intonation, phrasing, and emphasis is probably sufficient for us to favor the route via meanings since intonation, phrasing, and emphasis require understanding before they can be dubbed onto the text correctly. However, additional empirical evidence can be found in the small number of studies which have done cognitive analyses of the errors skilled readers make when reading continous text aloud.

Kolers (1966) had bilingual subjects read aloud passages made up of haphazardly alternating English and French words, for example, *His horse, followed de deux bassets, faisait la terre resonner under its even tread. Des gouttes* . . . Kolers found frequent translational errors in which subjects read, for example, *vent* as "wind," *hand* as "main," *of his* as "de sa," and *with* as "avec." These errors could only happen if readers recognized, say, the French word *vent* visually, accessed its meaning, then used the wrong (English) phonemic word production system thereby re- trieving the equivalent English word, "wind."

Semantic errors within a language were noted by Morton (1964c). His subjects were asked to read aloud passages which varied in their degree of approximation to natural English. A total of 133 errors were noted in which a word in the text was replaced in reading aloud by a word of equivalent or similar meaning (for example, *evening* read as "morning," *Sunday* as "Saturday," *might* as "may," and *came* as "gone"). Once again these errors suggest that the passage was decoded to meaning before being re-encoded into speech.

Substitutions of semantically related words in Kolers's (1966) and Morton's (1964c) experiments suggest that meaning is intimately involved in reading aloud. How come there is time between a reader seeing a word and then saying it for the extraction and integration of meaning to occur? Morton (1964c) noted, as others had before, that in reading aloud their eyes are typically not fixating the word they are articulating. Instead the eyes may be three or four words ahead of the voice. There is a gap in reading text between fixation and articulation known as the "eye-voice span" (see Gibson and Levin, 1975). There are times when an eye-voice span is essential. Try reading aloud the sentence, *The prince noticed that the princess had a tear in her dress and a tear in her eye.* The ambiguous homograph *tear* can only be pronounced correctly if the eyes run ahead of the voice as far as the disambiguating words *dress* and *eye*. As Buswell (1920, p.41) put it, the eye-voice span "allows the mind to grasp and interpret a large unit of meaning before the voice must express it." Sixty years on there is no reason to dispute this claim. That said, if reading aloud were done entirely via meaning one might expect more synonym substitutions. For example, *mat* and *rug* have virtually identical meanings, as do *bucket* and *pail*, and though one might occasionally misread *mat* as "rug" or *bucket* as "pail," one does not regularly do so. It is possible that simultaneously operating, low-level grapheme-phoneme conversion serves to prevent these errors, for example, by informing the speech production machinery that the initial sound of the spoken word for *mat* begins with a /m/ sound (cf., Newcombe and Marshall, 1980), but it is also possible that the direct connections between recognition and production units serve this error-preventing purpose. This could be done by priming appropriate phonemic word production units so that less semantic input is needed from the semantic system to activate a correct word than a synonym.

THE ROLE OF SOUND IN READING

We have argued so far that skilled readers identify familiar words visually, and that sound is only used when attempting to identify unfamiliar words. Somehow, though, we have to reconcile this claim with the fact that most people when they read will report the presence of an "inner voice" saying the words as they are read. What is the nature of this inner voice? Does it play any useful role in reading?

Let us begin by clarifying just where inner speech might lie with respect to the accessing of meaning from print. The voice we hear inside our heads as we read pronounces irregular words correctly. It assigns the correct pronunciations to homographs like *tear*, *row*, and *minute*, and it gives appropriate emphasis and intonation to what is being read. This implies that the inner voice is synthesized *after* the written words have been identified and understood. That is, inner speech would seem to follow comprehension rather than mediating it. In terms of the model shown in Figure 3.1 one might propose that in reading meanings are accessed via the visual word recognition system that pronunciations are then accessed via the phonemic word production system, and that what we experience as inner speech is the internal recycling of phonemic forms back through the auditory word recognition system using the loop we have already held to be involved in phonically mediated reading.

If the above characterization is correct, then it would seem that we could dispose of inner speech without loss to comprehension. When reading certain authors we may actually want to hear the sounds of the words, but for many purposes the meaning may be all we seek. Pintner (1913) reviewed the early work on inner speech in reading and concluded that "articulation during the reading process is a habit, which is not necessary for the process" and that "practice in reading without articulation tends to aid ordinary reading." Pinter's conclusions were based on the introspective reports of earlier writers and on some experiments which are fairly crude by modern standards. More recent work suggests the Pintner's conclusions may need to be modified.

Attempts have been made to disrupt inner speech by having subjects read while simultaneously saying "the, the, the . . . ," counting repetitively from one to six, or indulging in some other form of "concurrent articulation." Comprehension is then tested by requiring the subject to respond to a later sentence. Using this technique, Slowiaczek and Clifton (1980) found that concurrent articulation did not impair comprehension of individual words or concepts but did impair the ability to comprehend relations between words or concepts. Levy (1975; 1977) found that readers engaging in concurrent articulation found it harder to detect changes such as substitution of synonyms or swapping of sentence subject and object between a passage sentence and the test sentence.

Baddeley, Eldridge and Lewis (1981) note that these experiments involve a short-term memory component because subjects have to retain the elements of the passage in order to compare the test sentence. They argue that concurrent articulation may exert its effects because it disrupts memory rather than comprehension. Accordingly, their subjects made judgments about sentences as they read them. In Baddeley, Eldridge, and Lewis's Experiment I readers were instructed to detect anomalous words inserted into otherwise sensible sentences. When engaged in concurrent articulation the readers detected fewer anomalies but were no slower at responding to those they did detect. In Experiment II readers detected fewer experimenter-introduced reversals of adjacent words when subvocalizing than when silent though, again, those they did detect were responded to equally rapidly.

What are we to make of these results? Baddeley, Eldridge, and Lewis suggest that inner speech "may provide a very useful additional cue in detecting relatively subtle changes in the wording of text, particularly where changes of order are involved." Slowiaczek and Clifton (1980) propose that inner speech creates an acoustic code, thereby providing access to speech comprehension mechanisms. This means that text read with accompanying inner speech may give the reader two chances at comprehending it, rather as if one were hearing a story while at the same time following the text with one's eyes. The extra pass through the comprehension processes could explain the superior detection of text errors in Baddelely, Lewis, and Elridge's experiments, and may also explain why subvocalization increases as readers progress from simple to difficult passages (Sokolov, 1972).

The view of inner speech in reading which emerges sees inner speech as not essential to comprehension but as providing a useful, supplementary source of input to comprehension processes. This may be particularly useful in aiding the comprehension of relations between propositions or concepts, or the understanding of new and difficult ideas. However, as in most aspects of the processing of words in combinations, one gains the impression that, rather than being able to provide answers, cognitive psychologists are just beginning to formulate the right questions.

SUMMARY OF CHAPTER 5

Eye movements in natural reading are made up of rapid jerks called *saccades* punctuated by longer pauses called *fixations*. Despite the sensation of smooth movement the eyes are in fact still for ninety percent of the time when we read. The effective visual field at each fixation embraces some ten or twelve letters or spaces and is more extended to the right of the fixation point than to the left.

Sentence structure must be analyzed for text to be understood, but sentence structure is not always necessary. Broca's aphasics can understand many sentences despite being unable to utilize sentence structure. Sentence comprehension is a continuous, ongoing process in which knowledge of the world plays an important part. The products of comprehension may be abstract propositions partly extracted from the text and partly added by the reader's own processes of inference. The processes responsible for text understanding are probably not specific to reading but are common to both reading and speech comprehension.

The products of comprehension may be used by poorer readers to assist identification of the currently fixated word, but skilled readers may not do so. Recent evidence and argument goes against the long-held opinion that context aids word recognition and suggests instead that skilled readers are content to use rapid, efficient stimulus-driven processes to extract meaning from print. Reading text aloud appears to occur via the extraction of meaning, done as words are held within the eye-voice span, though grapheme-phoneme conversion or word-specific input-output connections may play a supplementary, error-preventing role. Finally, the inner speech which accompanies much of ordinary reading does not provide the initial access to meaning but may afford a useful second pass through the language comprehension processes.

6 Spelling and Writing

So far we have concentrated on the progression from print to meaning and to pronunciation—on reading, in other words. But literate adults are able to *create* written language as well. In this chapter we shall look at the psychological processes which make writing and spelling possible. Once again we shall restrict ourselves initially to skilled performance and its acquired disorders (known as the *acquired dysgraphias*), and defer consideration of the learning process and of developmental disorders until later chapters. As compared with the amount of research and thought devoted to reading, the psychology of writing has been neglected. There are signs, however, that the situation is improving (see, for example, Frith, 1980; Gregg and Steinberg, 1980; Hartley, 1980). Also many of the ideas developed to explain reading can be adapted to explain writing processes.

Most of the work done on producing written language has looked at spelling; that is, at how we are able to produce the correct letter string for a particular word, and what sorts of errors we make when we are incorrect. Work on acquired disorders of writing has also tended to focus on disorders of spelling. The contents of this chapter will inevitably reflect this concentration on spelling, but we will also look at theories of the production of written texts and sentences, and at how writing and reading might interrelate.

PLANNING TO WRITE

Compare the transcript of a casual conversation with a passage of text from a book and you will notice many differences. Typical speech has a simple grammatical structure though it often lacks clear sentence boundaries, is repetitive but rather inexplicit, is informal, and contains many pauses, ums, ers, and false starts. In contrast, typical writing has a more complex grammatical structure, clear sentence boundaries, is explicit, formal, and nonrepetitive. Faced with such differences one might be tempted to say that speech and writing use two quite different grammars, but as Leech, Deuchar, and Hoogenraad (1982) observe, there is really a continuum rather than a dichotomy between spoken and written language styles. The language used in a personal letter between close friends may be more "speechlike" than the speech of a lecture, formal discussion, or job interview. There are many different styles or "registers" of English, some more formal than others. Certainly typical writing tends more toward the formal end of the continuum than typical speech, but as we have seen the two overlap considerably.

That said, psychologists who have studied the higher-level aspects of writing—the production of sentences, paragraphs, and texts—have tended to concentrate on formal writing, for example, the composition of set essays by students. Flower and Hayes (1980) note that many texts on "how to write" divide the process up into three broad stages—Pre-Write, Write, and Rewrite. Pre-Write encompasses all the reading around, evaluating, and thinking which must be done before writing can begin. Flower and Hayes suggest that introducing writers to the notion of a pre-write phase can help remove some of the guilt often associated with "mulling over" or just gazing into space. However, they also argue that their experience of studying the writing process shows that pre-write, write, and rewrite are often intermingled operations rather than separate and discrete stages. This is also Wason's (1980) view. He notes that writers often comment to the effect that the act of writing helps clarify their thinking on a topic, and that new ideas often occur to them as they write. For instance, a historian observes that:

> One of the cheering things about writing is that it often clears my mind and stimulates ideas and directions of arguments which I had not thought of.

Another writer comments in similar vein that:

> Writing for me is an experience of knowing what to say. I can make endless schemes of how the piece should run but it never comes out according to plan. Until I have written a paragraph, I do not even know whether what I am saying is true. Once it is down in black and white I frequently see that it is not and then I have to ask myself why it is not. (Wason, 1980, p. 133)

The model of writing proposed by Hayes and Flower (1980) contains separate components but they are in continuous interaction rather than being a linear sequence of stages. In their model, the initial planning of writing is influenced by the task environment (such things as the topic to be written about and the intended audience) and by the writer's long-term memory which includes his or her knowledge of the topic, knowledge of the audience, and stored formulae or general plans for essay writing. Given this input one must set about planning the content of the essay, bearing in mind certain constraints and goals such as the requirements to make the text comprehensible, rememberable, persuasive, or enticing (see Collins and Gentner, 1980). Clearly these constraints will influence different writing assignments to different degrees. A thriller writer must be enticing and comprehensible but need not be especially rememberable while an office memo need only aim at comprehensibility.

In planning one must then organize the list of topics or ideas one wishes to mention into a logical order. According to Hayes and Flower this all takes place in a nonlinguistic conceptual code which must then be translated into language. The necessity for ideas and concepts to be originally represented in an abstract "language of thought"—the propositional "gist" of the previous chapter—can be appreciated if one reflects that many people can express the same ideas equally well in two or three different spoken languages, or that a series of instructions can often be conveyed as well, if not better, in a flow chart or series of pictures as in a series of sentences.

In Hayes's and Flower's model, each "idea" or "topic" must be broken down into a sequence of propositions which will be expressed in individual sentences or clauses. One then starts to write. Some writers formulate a very detailed plan before they start to write; others, as we have seen, have only the sketchiest of outlines in their heads and let the topics organize themselves as they write. Some writers continuously monitor and edit their prose for spelling, grammaticality, accuracy of meaning, and comprehensibility; others prefer to "get it all down" on paper first with minimal editing then set about improving the product when they prepare a subsequent draft.

A character in one of Molière's plays was surprised to discover that he had been talking prose all his life. While practice at writing may improve and hone the skills we have just discussed, there is nothing to suggest that they are in any way unique to the production of written language. These descriptions of planning, translating, executing, and monitoring must also characterize a story teller in an oral culture, a best man preparing a wedding speech, a dissatisfied customer preparing what to say to the shop manager tomorrow, a child preparing his or her "class news," or a student asked to talk at short notice on a debating proposition (as in the study by Butterworth, 1975). True, the fact that writing creates a permanent physical product may make it more amenable to critical editing and correcting, but it remains the case that the processes deployed in the production of texts and sentences are almost certainly part of our general language production competence, just as the processes deployed in text and sentence comprehension are part of our general language comprehension competence.

The point where speech and writing diverge is the point where we decide whether we are going to output our message as strings of phonemes (speech) or as strings of letters (writing). If it is strings of letters that we are concerned to produce, then in order to communicate effectively we must use those letter strings which convention recognizes as the "correct" spellings of the words we wish to use. Those are, after all, the spellings which our readers' visual word recognition units will be set up to identify. How are we able to produce correct spellings at least most of the time? That is the question to which we shall now turn our attention.

PHONIC MEDIATION OF SPELLING?

A cognitive psychologist seeking to create a model of spelling might be tempted to suggest that spelling is psychologically parasitic upon speaking. One could propose that a writer begins with the meaning of the word he or she wants to write then accesses the phonemic form from the phonemic word production system. The writer could then use his or her knowledge of phoneme-grapheme correspondences to create a spelling for the target word. What we have just outlined is, of course, a phonic mediation model for spelling, and such models seem to have been even more attractive as theories of spelling than as theories of reading. This is especially true among neuropsychologists; for example, we find the great Russian neuropsychologist A. R. Luria writing:

> Psychologically, the writing process involves several steps. The flow of speech is broken down into individual sounds. The phonemic significance of these sounds is identified and the phonemes represented by letters. Finally, the individual letters are integrated to produce the written word. (Luria, 1970, pp. 323–324)

Unfortunately, phonic mediation theories of spelling soon run aground against many of the same obstacles that caused the equivalent theories of reading to flounder.

Homophones and irregular words

Homophones are very common in English yet they create the same problems for phonic mediation theories of spelling as they create for equivalent theories of reading. The pronunciation of *won* is the same as *one*, *their* is the same as *there*, *rain* is the same as *rein* is the same as *reign*, and so on. The spelling of these words is determined by the meaning to be conveyed: a phonic mediation model like Luria's provides no mechanism for selecting the correct spelling of homophones. Even more seriously, it does not explain how we manage to avoid producing homophonic nonwords such as *RANE* for *rain* or *CASSEL* for *castle* (N.B. we are only considering here the spelling of familiar words by skilled writers).

Irregular or other words which are unpredictable in their spelling also create problems for any phonic mediation theory. No one who tries to assemble a spelling based on the pronunciation of "yacht" is likely to arrive at anything even approaching the correct spelling. Even apart from such out-and-out exception words, it is also the case that far fewer words are consistent, and therefore predictable, in the sound-to-print (spelling) direction than in the print-to-sound (reading) direction. Double *e* is consistently pronounced, so the pronunciation of a word like *street* is predictable from its spelling. However, if one knew only the pronunciation of "street" then its correct spelling might be *STREET*, but it could also be *STREAT* or *STRETE*. As Hatfield and Patterson (1983) note, there are only a comparatively few words such as *lunch*, *thing*, and *spent* which are predictable in the sense that one can hardly imagine them being spelled differently.

Phonological dysgraphia

If anyone is still not convinced that phonic mediation theories of spelling are not viable, we can cite neuropsychological evidence to support this verdict. Shallice (1981) reported a patient, P. R., who could spell correctly more than ninety percent of dictated real words but who could produce plausible spelling for hardly any nonwords. This was not because he could not hear or say the nonwords he was being asked to spell since he could repeat spoken nonwords without difficulty. He could also successfully read aloud a fair proportion of *written* nonwords. The dysgraphia, there-fore, was more or less specific to the process of assembling spellings phonically from pronunciations. Shallice calls this syndrome "phonologi-cal dysgraphia" because of its obvious similarity to phonological dyslexia. P. R. could not assemble spellings from sound yet could spell the great majority of words whose spellings he had learned before his stroke. This must imply a spelling mode or route which does not depend on phonic assembly procedures. What is needed is a mechanism by which spellings may be addressed in memory and retrieved as wholes.

ADDRESSED SPELLINGS

The alternative to phonically assembled spellings would seem to be addressed spellings; that is, spellings retrieved for some form of long-term store of learned spellings. Morton (1980) called this store the graphic output logogen system; we shall call it the *graphemic word production system*. Like its counterpart, the phonemic word production system, the graphemic word productions system is held to contain many individual production units; in fact, one for each word its possessor is able to spell.

When we are writing we start out with the meaning of a word we want to write—that is, with its semantic representation. Following Morton (1980) we shall argue that the semantic representation serves as input to the graphemic word production system where it will usually activate the appropriate and correct unit. That unit will in turn release the appropriate and correct letter string. Shallice's (1981) phonological dysgraphic patient retained his graphemic word production system though he had lost the capacity to assemble spellings phonically. The fact that he could still spell even highly predictable words like *lunch*, *thing*, and *spent* shows that the graphemic word production system stores *all* familiar spellings, not just those of irregular or unpredictable words.

Figure 6.1 shows a simple and preliminary model for this mode of spelling directly from meaning. When considering speech production we introduced the concept of a phonemic buffer as a short-term store capable of holding a word's phonemic representation in the interval between it being accessed and being articulated. Writing is slower than speaking, and there is need of an equivalent *graphemic buffer* capable of holding a word's spelling between retrieval and execution, and capable of maintaining the latter portion of a word while the earlier portion is being written. Such a buffer is therefore incorporated into Figure 6.1.

Deep dysgraphia

Phonological dysgraphia is not the only acquired dysgraphic syndrome in which the patient appears limited to addressed spellings with no capacity for assembling spellings from pronunciations. This pattern is also found in *deep dysgraphia* where, as might be expected, other symptoms also occur, the most noteworthy being semantic writing errors.

The deep dyslexic patient, G. R., studied by Marshall and Newcombe not only made semantic errors when reading (e.g., reading *gnome* as "pixie"), but also made semantic errors when attempting to spell words. For example, when asked to write "star" he wrote *MOON*, and when asked to write "bun" he wrote *CAKE* (Newcombe and Marshall, 1980).

Bub and Kertesz (1982) provide a more detailed report of a "deep dysgraphic." Their patient was twenty-one-year-old woman, J. C. (who should not be confused with Marshall and Newcombe's, 1973, surface dyslexic of the same initials). J. C. had suffered a stroke which left her

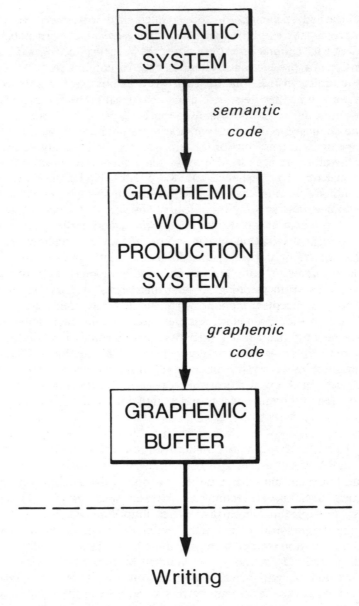

Figure 6.1 A model of addressed spelling.

with good comprehension of both spoken and written words, halting "telegraphic" speech, and poor writing. She made many semantic errors when writing words to dictation (e.g., "chair" written as *TABLE*, "time" as *CLOCK*, "yacht" as *BOAT*, and "give" as *TAKE*), was better at spelling concrete words than abstract words, was poorer on function words than nouns, and was very poor at writing nonwords to dictation. Though she could repeat nonwords aloud, J. C. was very poor at writing them and managed only 5/20 four-letter and 0/17 eight-letter nonwords. Her errors in this task sometimes took the form of writing a real word similar in sound to the dictated nonword (e.g., for "wabe" she wrote *WADE*, and for "besh" she wrote *BASH*). J. C. could even make semantic errors based on this strategy. For instance, asked to spell "blom" she wrote *FLOWER* (presumably via "bloom"), and asked to spell "lobinger" she wrote *OYSTER* (presumably via "lobster").

Newcombe and Marshall's deep dyslexic, G. R., also made derivational spelling errors (e.g., "tap" spelled as *TAPS*). Bub and Kertesz do not report such errors for J. C. but she may not have been asked to spell the sorts of words which would most lend themselves to derivational errors. In deep dysgraphia there would not appear to be any strict equivalent to the visual errors of deep dyslexics (here one would be looking for the patient producing real words similar in appearance rather than meaning to the dictated target word; for example "chair" misspelled as *CHOIR*).

The inability of deep dysgraphics to spell nonwords indicates a loss of the capacity for phonically assembled spelling. Their semantic errors and difficulty with abstract words suggest an additional impairment of the semantic system. Now, since there is no reason to believe that the same semantic system is not involved in both reading and spelling, it might be argued that deep dysgraphics should also be deep dyslexics; that is, they should make semantic errors in reading as well as in writing. G. R. did this, but J. C. did not—her reading was quite normal. Bub and Kertesz report that J. C. appeared unaware that she was producing a semantic error as she wrote but detected the error immediately after producing it, illustrating the potential of reading as an error-detecting check on writing (a point we shall return to later). In order to retain the notion of a single semantic system for both reading and writing we might propose that in J. C. the semantic system was intact (because she did not make semantic reading errors) but that the transmission of semantic codes to the graphemic word production system was in some way impaired.

A final point to observe is that J. C.'s deep dysgraphic symptoms disappeared within six months. Her ability to spell nonwords returned, she ceased to have problems with abstract words, and she stopped making semantic writing errors. Such rapid recovery is unlikely to have come about through relearning—it is more probable that her stroke had caused certain psychological processes to become *temporarily* inaccessible or inefficient. In contrast, G. R., for example, has remained deep dyslexic and deep dysgraphic for over thirty-five years with no sign of recovery.

Slips of the pen and addressed spellings

We have argued that our capacity to spell *there* and *their* correctly, or *piece* and *peace*, is evidence against obligatory phonic mediation theories of spelling. However, though we *usually* spell these homophones correctly, most readers will be familiar with the experience of intending to write *their* but inadvertently writing *there* instead. These errors are one of several different types of *slip of the pen* which skilled writers will make from time to time. They are not errors of knowledge caused by ignorance of a word's correct spelling, but are errors of performance caused by momentary derailments of the normally smooth-running cognitive processes which make writing possible. There are a number of insightful early papers on slips of the pen, notably Bawden (1900), Douse (1900), and Wells (1906), and in recent years some cognitive psychologists have again turned to studying these involuntary deviations from intended writing performance for the light they can shed on the underlying psychological processes (e.g., Ellis, 1979b; 1982c; Hotopf, 1980; Wing and Baddeley, 1980). We will examine other types of slip of the pen later, but for the moment we are concerned with the implications of homophone slips.

We cannot revert to the suggestion that phonemic forms alone are used to select spellings or homophone slips would be habitual rather than very occasional, but these errors seem to imply that the phonemic representations of words do play a part in the retrieval of spellings from the graphemic word production system. Morton (1980) suggests that the system receives *two* inputs—a semantic specification of the meaning of the word to be written from the semantic system, and a phonemic specification of the sound of the word to be written from the phonemic word system (Morton's speech output logogen systems). Clearly the phonemic form of "their" will activate the graphemic word production units for both *their* and *there* although only the unit for *their* will be receiving a semantic input. We can explain homophone errors and near-homophone errors like *SURGE* for *search* or *COULD* for *good* if we assume that, just occasionally, a phonemic form may activate the graphemic word production unit for an incorrect word similar or identical in sound to the target word.

A small number of semantic errors also occur as slips of the pen, for example writing *SPEAKING* for *reading* or *LAST WEEK* for *next week* (Ellis, 1979c; Hotopf, 1980). These errors may occur when a semantic input to the graphemic word production system activates the wrong unit. The scarcity of these errors in writing as compared with speech may be due to the fact that the phonemic input to the graphemic word production system will usually inhibit the production of words similar in meaning but different in sound to the intended target word.

The sort of model of how skilled writers retrieve from memory the spellings of familiar words which arises from these considerations is shown in Figure 6.2. In the model the processes responsible for the

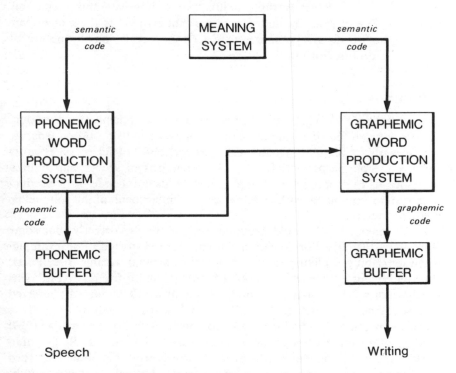

Figure 6.2 A more complete model of the retrieval of the addressed spellings of familiar words.

production of written and spoken words are partially distinct but closely interconnected. Thus, the same semantic system formulates the meanings of words whether they are to be written or spoken, but letter strings (graphemic forms) and pronunciations (phonemic forms) are retrieved from two separate word production systems, rather than being two outputs of a single system. Nevertheless, phonemic forms provide a supplementary input to the graphemic word production system, which may go some way towards explaining why when we are writing we also seem to be simultaneously talking to ourselves. (There are times in writing when this talk is necessary; for example, we chose between *a* and *an* on the basis of the initial *sound* of the following word rather than its initial letter—compare *a habit* versus *an hour*).

One might at this point ask whether the graphemic word production system, like the visual word recognition system, and the phonemic word production system is not in actuality a morphemically based system. Evidence that it might be comes from derivational slips of the pen such as writing *RELATING* instead of *relative* or *DISCUSSING* instead of *discussion* (Ellis, 1979c; Hotopf, 1980). As yet, however, this is the only pertinent piece of evidence and alternative explanations of these errors are possible, so we should perhaps return an open verdict on the nature of graphemic production units.

Patient R. D.

One advantage of having separate phonemic and graphemic word production systems within one's model is that it allows one to postulate separate impairments of the two systems. Ellis, Miller, and Sin (in press) recently studied an aphasic patient, R. D., whose patterns of speech and writing errors led us to propose a mild impairment of his graphemic word production system combined with a more severe impairment of his phonemic word production system.

In his speech R. D. could pronounce many words correctly, but some words—particularly less common words—were distorted. For example, when describing a picture depicting activities around a camp fire, R. D. called a stream a "stringt," a stool a "strow," and a fire a "fiyest." His errors were not consistent; within the space of a few minutes he referred to a scout as a "skat," a "skirt," and a "skrut." Analysis of R. D.'s mispronunciations in speaking led us to concur with Butterworth's (1979) account of a similar (though more severe) case and argue that R. D. could retrieve the full phonemic forms of many words from his phonemic word production system, but that on some occasions, particularly when searching for a less common word, he could only retrieve part of its phonemic form and constructed an attempt at the word based on that information. Thus, he seems to have known that "scout" begins with /sk/, ends with /t/, and has one central vowel, but seems to have been unable to retrieve the information specifying what that vowel is.

To come to the point about spelling, R. D. was often able to write a word he could not say correctly. For instance, he correctly wrote the word *penguin* while calling it a "senstenz," and he correctly wrote the word *elephant* while calling it an "enelust" or "keneltun." R. D. cannot have been spelling via phoneme-grapheme correspondences since (a) his pronunciations were often incorrect and (b) he could spell irregular words as well as he could spell regular ones. R. D.'s speech problems were not of a peripheral articulatory nature since he could pronounce long and articulatory complex words provided they were common words he had used many times.)

R. D.'s spellings must have been originating from his graphemic word production system (indeed his pattern of deficits and abilities provides further evidence for the existence of such a system). His writing was not, however, totally unimpaired. Table 6.1 shows a selection of R. D.'s spelling errors made when trying to write picture names. Very few of the errors could be described as "phonetic"; that is, *sounding* like the target

TABLE 6.1
Errors made by patient R. D. when spelling picture names

TARGET WORD	ERROR	TARGET WORD	ERROR
snowman	SCOWMAN	leopard	LEOPALD
basket	BASHEL	celery	CELEBRA
sledge	SEDGE	kangaroo	KENGABA
thumb	THUNB	salt	CALT
clown	COLOWN	scissors	SICESSE
giraffe	GARFARA	squirrel	SIGIL

word. Of particular interest are errors like *SICESSE* for *scissors* and *THUNB* for *thumb* where R. D. included a silent letter in his attempt (the *c* and the *b* in these cases), and also errors like *GARFARA* for *giraffe* and *CELABRA* for *celery* where R. D. correctly used the rather unpredictable initial *g* and *c* where *j* and *s* might be expected.

R. D.'s spelling errors suggest that, rather like his pronunciation errors, they arise as a consequence of having only partially retrieved the word's full specification. This implies that retrieval of words from the graphemic word production system is not all-or-nothing, but that on occasions an attempt at the spelling of a word may be based on partial information about the graphemic form of a word. We shall see later that the concept of partial retrieval of information from the graphemic word production system is also necessary to explain some of the spelling errors made by normal children and adults, and also by developmental dyslexics.

TOWARD A COMPOSITE MODEL FOR ADDRESSED AND ASSEMBLED SPELLINGS

Logical problems with obligatory phonic mediation theories and neuropsychological analyses of phonological dyslexia and deep dyslexia support the view that normal writers retrieve the spellings of familiar words from some form of graphemic word production system. Nevertheless, the existence of *optional* processes capable of assembling spellings from pronunciations is indisputable and clearly demonstrated by asking people to produce a plausible spelling for a dictated nonword, or to think of alternative ways of spelling a familiar word (e.g., *MUNE* for "moon," or *CHARE* for "chair"). This route is, of course, available to us if we wish to assemble a plausible candidate spelling of a word whose pronunciation we know but whose spelling we are unsure of.

Analogies and correspondences in assembled spellings

How *do* adults assemble spellings for unfamiliar words? In particular, do they make use of analogies with similar sounding familiar words? Campbell (1983) has provided evidence that skilled writers *do* use analogies when assembling spellings. She adapted a task used by Kay and Marcel (1981) who, it will be remembered, showed that one can influence how normal subjects will pronounce a nonword like *yead* by preceding it with either *bead* or *head*. Campbell dictated words and nonwords to normal subjects and showed that they would tend to spell a nonword like "prein" as *PRAIN* if they had recently spelled the word "brain," but as *PRANE* if they had recently spelled "crane." This implies that adult subjects are using analogies to assemble spellings for a new words, and that the particular analogy used can be influenced by familiar words recently heard.

How is analogical spelling to be explained in terms of a model like the one shown in Figure 6.2? The phonemic form of an unfamiliar word or nonword like "prein" might be transmitted to the graphemic word production system along the route from the phonemic buffer that we introduced to account for homophonic slips of the pen like writing *there* instead of *their*. At the graphemic word production system the phonemic form will activate the production units of similar sounding familiar words like *pray*, *brain*, and *crane*. If, as in Campbell's (1983) experiment, one has recently written either *BRAIN* or *CRANE* then the primed production unit is the one most likely to contribute to the candidate spelling. However, one does not write either *BRAIN* or *CRANE*; there must exist processes of *graphemic assembly* capable of isolating and combining only the relevant portions of activated words. Unfortunately we can as yet say very little about the operation of this graphemic assembly system.

Although analogies will offer themselves for many new words, others may not lend themselves so readily to spelling by analogy. In such cases writers trying to assemble a plausible spelling may resort to breaking the phonemic form of the unfamiliar word down into syllables or even single phonemes and applying low-level phoneme-grapheme correspondences. For example, you may have heard the name of the Russian psychologist *Pavlov* used in a lecture and want to use it yourself in a essay. You could, of course, go looking for the correct spelling in an appropriate book, but you may instead opt to assemble a plausible spelling according to how the name sounds. *Pavlov* is a somewhat unusual name for which no analogies may present themselves. To spell it you must first *segment* the phonemic form of the word into its component consonant and vowel *sounds* (phonemes). You must then supply the appropriate letter for each phoneme (or letter group in cases like *th*, *sh*, *oo*, and *ee*) and assemble those letters into a candidate spelling. If the target word is *Pavlov*, which happens to be one of the minority of words containing predictable phoneme-grapheme correspondences, then your assembled candidate spelling has a good chance of being correct.

In spelling by low-level correspondences we can, therefore, distinguish at least three operations. First, the phonemic form of the word to be spelled must be segmented into its component syllables or phonemes. Second, the letters which commonly represent those sound segments must be supplied. Third, the letters must be assembled into a candidate spelling. Presumably this graphemic assembly stage employs the same processes as are used when spellings are being assembled by analogy. The resultant candidate spelling will then be deposited in the graphemic buffer ready for writing.

We have now outlined all the component processes that a model of skilled spelling would seem to require. Figure 6.3 shows the way they are thought to fit together. The fact that we can repeat nonwords which we hear and which can have no entries in our auditory word recognition or phonemic word productions systems, means that there must be some connection between the acoustic analysis system and the phonemic buffer

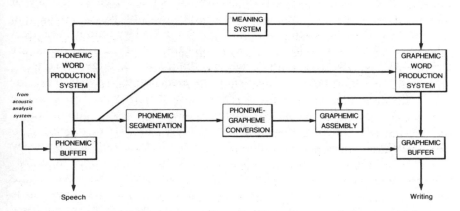

Figure 6.3 A model for both addressed and assembled spelling.

which bypasses the word recognition and production systems. This connection also permits the model to explain our ability to attempt spellings for dictated nonwords. Once again, this model is only meant as a visual aid to supplement a fuller description of how the individual components are thought to operate. If the model has a virtue it is in the way it lays out all of the components simultaneously and perhaps facilitates the appreciation of possible interrelations between components and the realization that in a complex system many things can be happening at many different places at the same time.

APPLYING THE MODEL

Having built our model of spelling we now need to test it in use. To do that we shall look at the sorts of spelling errors made by skilled writers, at individual differences among skilled writers, and at further varieties of acquired dysgraphia.

Spelling errors

Normal writers make two fundamentally different sorts of errors when trying to write a word. First, you may know full well how a word should be written but inadvertently omit some letters, or misorder them, or even write quite the wrong word. We are all prone to these lapses of execution which are known as slips of the pen, and we shall examine them more closely later for the light they can shed on writing processes. The second and perhaps more commonplace type of error arises when a writer does not in fact know the correct spelling of a word and makes an incorrect attempt to write it. These spelling errors are errors of knowledge which happen when the graphemic form of a word is not stored completely or correctly in a writer's graphemic word production system. Wing and Baddeley (1980) examined the errors made by secondary school candidates applying for entrance to Cambridge colleges. Most of the errors are phonic errors which, when pronounced, sound like the target word (e.g., RESURECT for resurrect, PLEBIAN for plebeian, ENDOCHRINE for endocrine). Similarly, Sloboda (1980) reports that fifty out of fifty-five errors produced by university students and staff were phonic (e.g., PUMMICE for pumice, REBLE for rebel, and DIRTH for dearth). Evidence for the use of analogies may be present in the Wing and Baddeley corpus. For example, one candidate detected the word proper in propaganda and spelled it PROPERGANDA. The candidate who wrote REKNOWNED for renowned appears to have believed that renowned is related to know and so included the unpronounced k. Another candidate wrote *UNWRAVELLED* for *unravelled*, apparently by analogy with *unwrapped*.

It will be recalled that the patient R. D. seemed sometimes to be able to retrieve only part of a word's spelling and built his attempt at the word around that skeleton. Similar things may be detected in the spelling errors of normal adults. For example, undergraduate students studied by Baron, Trieman, Wilf, and Kellman (1980) produced errors such as *COLORNEL* and *COLNEL* for *colonel*, *RHYTHEM* and *RHYTHUM* for *rhythm*, *PNEWMONIA* and *PNEMONIA* for *pneumonia*. These students knew that *colonel* has a silent *l* in it somewhere, that *rhythm* contains a silent *h* and a *y* where an *i* might be expected, and that *pneumonia* begins with a silent *p*. That is, these students possessed partial information about the spellings of these words which they then fleshed out with analogies (cf., the *new* in *PNEWMONIA*) or grapheme-phoneme correspondences.

In sum, skilled writers will quite often possess some information about the spelling of at least parts of a word whose total spelling they are unsure of. This partial knowledge, when present, is supplemented by procedures for converting phonemic forms into letter strings. These procedures will probably operate on the principle of the largest available phonemic unit, will use analogies where available, but can resort to correspondences between individual phonemes and letters or letter groups where necessary.

Individual differences

Even among literate adults there would seem to be individual differences in the extent to which a person will rely on assembled or addressed spelling. Baron, Trieman, Wilf, and Kellman (1980) asked students to generate as many acceptable respellings as they could for a set of eight familiar words (e.g, *rye* could be respelled as *RI*, *RHI*, *WRIGH*, and so on, but not as *RIAGH* or *WREA*). This is rather like Baker's (1980) spelling reform task which was mentioned in Chapter 1 and is clearly a test of phoneme-grapheme conversion ability. Students differed considerably on how many acceptable respellings they could create. Eighteen of the best respellers formed the "Phoenecian" group and sixteen of the worst respellers formed the "Chinese" group. The two groups were then asked to spell some regular and some irregular words. They did not differ on the total number of errors made, but the Phoenecian group made a greater proportion of "phonetic errors." In particular they tended to spell irregular words as if they were regular.

There are certain problems with the criteria used to distinguish between Chinese and Phoenecians in this study (Ellis, 1982c), but it seems likely, nevertheless, that people differ in the ease with which they can establish the graphemic word production units which will enable them to address whole spellings in memory at a later date, and they also differ in their capacity to assemble acceptable letter strings from phonemic forms. Most adults are probably either good or mediocre at both these skills, but there may exist a minority who are good at spelling from memory but poor at spelling from sound (true "Chinese") and a complementary minority who are good at spelling from sound but poor at spelling from memory (true "Phoenecians"). We shall see in Chapter 8 that these two dimensions of individual difference are also relevant to understanding the spelling of developmental dyslexics.

Surface dysgraphia

Beauvois and Dérousné (1981) described a French patient (initials R. G.) who could readily produce a plausible spelling in response to a spoken nonword but who made many errors when trying to spell real words which would have caused him no difficulties before his stroke. His spelling errors to real words were always phonic; that is, they would sound like the target word if read aloud. Because R. G. always spelled phonically, he was more likely to be correct when attempting to spell regular words than irregular ones.

Beauvois and Dérousné coined the term "lexical dysgraphia" to describe R. G.'s condition. Hatfield and Patterson (1983) prefer the term "phonological spelling" when referring to their similar English patient (T. P.), whereas the name which we shall use, "surface dysgraphia," highlights the similarity with surface *dyslexia* which we met in Chapter 4. Surface *dyslexics* have an impaired visual word recognition system and consequently are obliged to rely heavily on the phonic reading route. Surface *dysgraphics* appear to have an impaired graphemic word production system and therefore are obliged to use the phoneme to grapheme conversion system when trying to spell. The hallmark of phoneme to grapheme conversion is, of course, the "phonic" spelling error. Examples from Hatfield and Patterson's patient T. P. include "nephew" spelled as *NEFFUE*, "biscuit" as *bisket*, and "subtle" as *SUTTEL*.

As one would expect, T. P. was more likely to spell a regular word correctly than an irregular one. However, as with surface dyslexics, whole-word mechanisms were not completely destroyed. T. P. managed to spell correctly on at least one occasion quite a number of irregular words, including *cough, sign, aunt*, and *answer*; such spellings could only have come from the graphemic word production system. Although Patterson and Hatfield did not study this directly, it appears to have been the higher frequency words which T. P. could still spell correctly.

When T. P. misspelled a word her errors sometimes demonstrated that she had partial information about the word's correct spelling. Examples include "borough" spelled as *PUROUGH*, "sword" as *SWARD*, and "yacht" as *YHAGT*. The point here is that the *-ough* in *PUROUGH*, the *w* in *SWARD*, and the *h* and *a* in *YHAGT* are all difficult or impossible to predict on the basis of phoneme-grapheme conversion however that conversion is achieved. It appears that, like R. D., T. P. could not always retrieve a word's spelling in full from her graphemic word production system but could sometimes retrieve *part* of its spelling; this partial specification was then supplemented by phonic processes to produce the attempted spelling. However, in the case of *NEFFUE*, *BISKET*, and *SUTTEL* even this partial knowledge deserted her and her attempts were purely phonic (but note that *SUTTEL* is quite close to *sutil*, the original spelling of *subtle* before it was "reformed").

A final feature of T. P.'s spelling is that she sometimes misspelled a word dictated in a disambiguating context as its homophone. Thus she spelled "sale" as *SAIL*, "write" as *RIGHT*, and "sum" as *SOME*. Now, *right* and *some* are themselves irregular words so these spellings could not have been assembled phonically. What seems to happen is that when the correct spelling of a word is inaccessible, the phonemic form sometimes activates the spelling of a homophone. (N.B. We have argued earlier that phonemic codes are used in conjunction with semantic codes to retrieve spellings from the graphemic word production system.)

Surface dysgraphia is quite a complex syndrome, so I shall summarize the main features with particular reference to Hatfield's and Patterson's patient T. P.

1. T. P. has lost access to the production units for less common words in her graphemic word production systems.
2. If T. P. *can* retrieve a word's spelling in full she obviously writes the word correctly. However, when the full specification is not available she may still be able to retrieve part of the word's spelling: *SWARD* and *YHAGT* are examples of misspellings based on partial knowledge.
3. Alternatively, if a word's spelling is inaccessible, the spelling of a more common homophone may be retrieved. This implies that phonemic forms are used in conjunction with meanings to select appropriate spellings.
4. As a last resort T. P. will attempt to assemble a candidate spelling for the word on the basis of its pronunciation using low-level phoneme-grapheme correspondences. This strategy results in phonic errors like *NEFFUE* for "nephew."

Amnestic dysgraphia

Surface dysgraphics have an impaired "direct" spelling route and consequently rely heavily on the phonic route. Phonological dysgraphics have an impaired phonic route but can still spell by the direct route. What if both routes are incapacitated through brain injury? This is what appears to have happened in the case of a patient described by Bastian (1869) whose syndrome Bastian called "amnestic dysgraphia." The patient had only slight problems in speaking but his attempts to write words resulted in sequences of random (though well-formed) letters. Klein (1951) described a similar and, if anything, purer case. These patients appear to have lost the ability to convert meanings or sounds into spellings either directly from the graphemic word production system or phonically via pronunciations. Thus they combine the deficits of both surface dysgraphia and phonological dysgraphia. However, amnestic dysgraphics still know the shapes of letters and can execute them proficiently.

FROM GRAPHEMES TO MOVEMENTS

Any normal person who knows how to spell a word can spell it aloud or re-arrange wooden alphabet blocks to form the word, or can write it in capital letters, in neat, lower-case print or in hasty, scribbled handwriting. That person may also be able to type the word, write it backwards in mirror writing like Leonardo da Vinci in his notebook, or for that matter enscribe the word in sand on the beach with the toes of his or her left foot. What all this goes to show is that whatever the graphemic code is, it is *not* a simple description of, say, the movements typically made when writing a particular word. A graphemic code must be capable of being executed in each of the above ways and must therefore be a comparatively abstract description of the letter sequence which constitutes a word's spelling. This is true whether that code is retrieved as a whole from the graphemic word production system or is assembled phonically.

Valenstein and Heilman (1979) describe a patient who after brain injury retained a good memory, good speech production and comprehension, good reading aloud, and good understanding of what he read. When a word was spoken to him he could spell it aloud correctly. He could also type reasonably well (he had never been skilled at typing). What he could *not* do was *write* of his own accord. Though he might be able to spell a word aloud or type it, his attempts to write it resulted in meaningless squiggles. This patient could retrieve graphemic codes from his graphemic word production system, as attested by his ability to spell words aloud or type them, but he appears to have lost the memory of the shapes of letters or the movements necessary to form them.

It seems likely that, once a graphemic code has been retrieved or assembled, the next step in the progression towards writing the word is to select the particular letter *shapes* which are to be used. An obvious factor is whether one is writing in CAPITAL (UPPER-CASE) LETTERS or small (lower-case) letters. However, many people use more than two versions of some letters. I, for example, use F and f when printing or writing neatly but will also use ϶ and ∮ in more casual writing. Similarly, I use *s* at the beginnings of words and more generally in neat handwriting, but I also use ∽ in casual writing, particularly within and at the ends of words.

So various factors combine in the decision as to which letter shapes will be used, but those shapes still have to be executed. Handwritten letters are constructed from combinations of strokes and the writer must know how to assemble these. I for one do not always form the same letter in the same way; for instance my *o* when written in isolation is usually done with an anticlockwise stroke, but when situated in a word like ᴍᴏᴏɴ the movement is in a clockwise direction.

Having decided on shapes and strokes and directions, the next decision concerns *size* of writing, because size determines which groups of muscles in the body are called into play in the attempt to write a word. Large writing, for example with chalk on a blackboard, involves movements of the shoulder and elbow joints, whereas those joints will be little used in writing a letter to a friend in normal, cursive handwriting. In the latter case it is the muscles which move the wrist and finger joints that must do the work.

Fortunately one does not have to make all these decisions consciously. As with the construction of sentences and the selection of words, it is usually sufficient to set the processes into operation and the rest happens without one having any conscious access whatsoever to the underlying processes. Often enough we only become aware that any mental processes are going on at all when they let us down. This may be a serious breakdown as in a developmental or acquired dysgraphia, or the sort of momentary lapse which results in a slip of the pen. Some slips of the pen are attributable to the letter level in the planning of writing rather than the word level. An analysis of these errors supports (or at least is compatible with) the theory of a progression from an abstract graphemic code to letter shapes, then to motor patterns, and finally to execution as a sequence of strokes (Ellis, 1982c).

For instance, writers will sometimes inadvertently anticipate a letter from a forthcoming word and include it in the word currently being written, for example, wanting to write *are not read* but writing *are rot read* instead. What happens if the anticipated letter moves from a position where it would be written as a small (lower-case) letter into a position where the intended, corrected letter would have been a capital (upper-case) letter? Wells (1906, pp. 90–91) reports just such a slip. He intended to write *The distribution* but anticipated the *d* of *distribution* to the beginning of *The* and in fact wrote *Dhe*. A corpus of my own slips includes other similar examples (Ellis, 1979b). These errors are explicable if what is anticipated is an abstract grapheme prior to the decision being made as to which *form* of the grapheme is appropriate (whether *d* or *D*, *G* or *g*, etc.).

A second type of slip involves the omission of a letter which occurs more than once in a word (e.g., writing *UNUSAL* for *UNUSUAL*, *inital* for *initial*, or *erros* for *errors*). In my corpus these errors all involve identical forms of the same letter which suggests that they occur after letter shapes have been specified; that is, at a stage in the production of writing after the stage at which anticipations of letters between words occur. Several other sorts of letter-level slips of the pen occur, and careful study of them can shed light on what goes on between knowing the letters of which a word is made and actually forming the correct sequence of strokes to create the pattern of lines on paper that is writing.

We have already seen in the patient described by Valenstein and Heilman (1979) that brain injury may cause an acquired dysgraphia in which the problem may lie in the transition from graphemes to movements. That is, the patient may know how a word should be spelled but may be unable to write it despite having no other more general problems with the control of his writing hand. Rosati and de Bastiani (1979) report a patient whose reading and speech were entirely normal but whose writing contained numerous omissions, reversals, and repetitions of letters, and also repetitions of letter strokes. Importantly, however, he could spell words orally without error (P. de Bastiani, personal communication, 1982). This shows that he could retrieve the graphemic forms of words, and that his problems lay in converting graphemic forms into handwriting (his control of his writing hand for other uses was unimpaired).

So, writing is subject to many different forms of acquired disorder, just as speech and reading are. Some disorders affect the patient's ability to address or assemble a spelling; other disorders affect the ability to execute the letter string as writing. However, all the acquired dysgraphias seem explicable in terms of impairment to one or more of the components of models of normal writing.

THE RELATIONSHIP BETWEEN WRITING AND READING

As we write we are also creating something we ourselves can read, either immediately or at some later date. Although we have tended so far to treat writing and reading as if they were quite separate and unrelated skills, in reality they must be much more intimately related. We probably detect many of our slips of the pen visually as soon as we have written them. People will also often say that if they are unsure of the spelling of a word it sometimes helps to write down alternatives and see which one *looks* right. Tenney (1980) has produced some evidence for the efficacy of this strategy.

At a higher level we may also reread what we have written to assess its grammaticality or its coherence. Anyone who does any significant amount of writing, whether it be essays, stories, poems, scientific papers, or company reports, knows that something which felt fluent and coherent as it was being written can seem stilted, disorganized, verbose, or pompous when reread after a few days or weeks. Once we have externalized our thoughts in writing we can then bring the same critical faculties to bear on our own creation as we would bring to bear on someone else's.

An aspect of the interrelationship between writing and reading concerns the question of whether they are mediated by distinct psychological processes, or whether in going from meaning to print we simply engage in reverse direction the same processes that we utilize in going from print to meaning. For example, is the graphemic word production system from which we retrieve the spellings of familiar words just the visual word recognition system operating in reverse? Allport (1982) and Allport and Funnell (1981) argue that it is: their scheme includes a single "orthographic lexicon" which translates between letter codes and meanings in both directions. Other psychologists such as Morton (1980) prefer to regard input and output as the responsibility of separate cognitive systems. To be frank there is as yet no data which compels the theorist to choose one way or the other between these alternatives, but there is at least one line of evidence which could turn out to be important.

Simultaneous writing and reading

Gertrude Stein (1874–1946) is best remembered as a poet, critic, patron of the arts, and author of such works as *Three Lives* and *The Autobiography of Alice B. Toklas*. Less widely known is the fact that in her early life she planned to become a psychologist, studied under William James, one of the founding fathers of the subject, and conducted various experiments. Some of these, carried out in collaboration with Leon M. Solomons, are reported in the pages of the *Psychological Review*, Volume 3, for 1896 (Solomons and Stein, 1896). Of special interest here is an experiment in which Solomons and Stein themselves practiced writing words to spoken dictation while at the same time reading a story silently for meaning. "At first," they tell us, "the subject is entirely unable to follow what he is reading. He reads, but does not get the meaning." However, "one very quickly gets sufficiently accustomed to the experiment to follow the story . . . [and] in a few hours' practice one is able to read his story with perfect ease and comfort, undisturbed by the constant interruptions for writing" (pp. 497–498). With still more practice, "The writing becomes non-voluntary. We hear the word, and we know we have written; that is all. . . . Every once in a while the story grows interesting, and we return to ourselves with a start to find that we have been going on writing just the same. . . . We suddenly become aware that our hand is writing something" (pp. 498–500).

There is much that is of interest in Solomons's and Stein's account, but what concerns us here is not so much what it felt like to read and write at the same time as the fact that it is possible to perform these two skills simultaneously at all. In a more recent and more rigorous replication of the Solomons and Stein study, Spelke, Hirst, and Neisser (1976) have shown that it is possible to read silently with understanding and at the same time write words to dictation without loss of efficiency to either task.

One can perform two tasks simultaneously without detriment to either provided that they do not compete for the same physical or mental processes. This applies, for example, to walking and talking, or even playing the piano from music by sight while simultaneously repeating speech heard through headphones (see Allport, 1980, for a review of such studies). Arguably it should not be possible to both read and spell at the same time, without loss of efficiency to either if the two tasks require the same mental lexicon to function in two opposite directions at once. However, if reading occupies a visual word recognition system while writing occupies a separate graphemic word production system, then the two tasks could happily co-exist. That said, the issue is not settled and the reader should keep an open mind on this topic (as on all).

THE RELATIONSHIP BETWEEN ACQUIRED DYSLEXIA AND ACQUIRED DYSGRAPHIA

The separation of acquired dyslexia from acquired dysgraphia, while useful for explanatory purposes, may have given the misleading impression that patients are either dyslexic or dysgraphic but seldom both. This is definitely not the case; injuries to the brain which impair writing tend also to impair reading. That said, some of the more peripheral visual dyslexias quite often occur without any dysgraphia, and some of the more peripheral motor dysgraphias quite often occur without any dyslexic difficulties. Indeed, we have already seen that deep dysgraphia which is definitely not a peripheral motor problem can occur without dyslexia. Even when a central dyslexia co-exists with a central dysgraphia in the same individual the reading and writing problem need not be simple complements of one another. We shall illustrate something of how dyslexia and dysgraphia may intermesh by considering one well-documented case study (R. G.) and one well-documented syndrome (letter-by-letter reading).

Patient R. G.

The alert reader might just have noticed the coincidence of initials (R. G.) between one of the phonological dyslexics described in Chapter 4 and one of the surface dysgraphics described earlier in this chapter. In fact there is no coincidence at all because these two R. G.'s are one and the same person. R. G. was an agricultural machinery sales manager who underwent brain surgery at the age of sixty-two. On recovery it was found that he could *read* virtually any familiar real word but very few nonwords (i.e., he was a phonological dyslexic). This implies an intact visual-semantic reading route via visual word recognition system but impaired letter-to-phoneme conversion. In marked contrast R. G. could readily *spell* nonwords to dictation, but his spelling of real words was predominantly "phonic" (and therefore sometimes correct for regular words but rarely so for irregular ones). This "surface dysgraphic" spelling pattern implies an impaired semantic-graphemic route via a graphemic word production system but intact phoneme-to-grapheme conversion. Thus we can see intact visual-to-semantic reading with impaired phonic reading co-existing alongside intact phonic spelling with impaired semantic-to-graphemic spelling in one and the same person. We shall see in later chapters that this pattern recurs in developmental contexts also.

Letter-by-letter reading

Patterson and Kay (1983) report four patients who showed the phenomenon of "letter-by-letter reading." In this long-established syndrome patients are unable to identify words as wholes, but instead work through each word from left to right identifying each letter separately and often naming each letter aloud. Letters are named rather than sounded; for example "double-u, aitch, aye, tee" for *what*. When the patient has reached the end (or nearly the end) of the word, he or she names it. Because words are processed letter-by-letter the time taken to identify a word increases as the number of letters in the word increases. Writing is always relatively intact in letter-by-letter readers, hence its alternative name of "alexia without agraphia."

The possible significance of the relatively well-preserved writing of letter-by-letter readers is also the reason why the syndrome is being treated here rather than in the earlier chapter on the acquired dyslexias. Warrington and Shallice (1980) propose that in letter-by-letter readers the visual word recognition system (what they call the "visual word-form system") has been destroyed but that the patient reads by using his or her spelling system. The idea is that as the patient identifies each letter of a word he or she builds up a graphemic code which can then access, in reverse direction, the graphemic word production system and the phoneme-grapheme conversion processes.

Evidence supporting this interpretation comes from the fact that although spelling is always reasonably good in letter-by-letter readers it is not always perfect. Specifically, two of the four letter-by-letter readers reported by Patterson and Kay (1983) were also surface dysgraphics. In fact one of them is the patient T. P. discussed at length earlier. Now, when T. P. attempted to read a word she would quite often identify the letters correctly but go on to misname the word, and her errors were just like those a surface dyslexic would make (e.g., *ache* pronounced as "aitch," *city* as "kitty," and *sword* pronounced with a /w/). On the Warrington and Shallice (1980) account such errors are to be expected since the patient is trying to read by the reverse use of a spelling system which is itself impaired.

It might be thought that there is no counterpart in normal adults to this rather odd strategy adopted by letter-by-letter readers (assuming the above account is correct). However, normal adults possess the rather peculiar ability to identify words whose letters are named aloud. For example, I can say "Y...A...C...H...T" and you will be able to say "yacht." Letter-by-letter readers can also identify words from oral spelling. It is possible that the only route to meaning available to letter-by-letter readers is also the route normal people use to identify orally spelled words. Quite how this route works and why it exists remains something of a mystery.

SUMMARY OF CHAPTER 6

Planning to write probably utilizes the same language production processes as speech production, though writing tends to have its own style and vocabulary. Writing is less interactive than natural speaking, but affords more opportunities for editing and amending; it probably diverges from speech at the point where word spellings must be accessed.

Skilled writers retrieve the spellings of familiar words as wholes from a graphemic word production system. A word is addressed by a combination of a semantic and a phonemic specification. Writers also possess a knowledge of analogies and/or phoneme-grapheme correspondences which enables them to assemble a plausible spelling for an unfamiliar word. Even among reasonably skilled writers there would seem to be individual differences in the extent to which a person will rely on addressed or assembled spelling.

The phonological dysgraphic P. R. could still retrieve the spellings of familiar words from his graphemic word production system but had lost the ability to assemble spellings piecemeal from their phonemic forms. Deep dysgraphics also rely exclusively on addressed spellings, but make semantic errors in the retrieval process. Surface dysgraphics, in contrast, rely heavily on phonically assembled spellings, having lost the ability to access the spellings of many familiar words from their graphemic word production systems.

Patient R. D used addressed spellings but was often only able to retrieve part of the word's spelling and constructed an attempt at the target based on that partial information. Some of the spelling errors made by skilled writers also appear to be based on the retrieval from memory of part of a word's spelling, supplemented perhaps by phoneme-grapheme conversion.

Whether spellings are addressed or assembled, the original graphemic code must be a relatively abstract one capable of being output as oral spelling, typing, upper-case print, cursive handwriting, etc. If writing is the chosen output mode, then it is proposed that the first step involves the selection of letter shapes, that the second step involves the selection of the motor patterns necessary to execute the chosen letter shapes, and that the third and final step involves realizing the motor patterns as sequences of strokes. Different letter-level slips of the pen seem attributable to different stages in this progression from abstract graphemes to coordinated physical movements. Brain injury can affect the transition from graphemes to movements without impairing the patient's knowledge of the correct spellings of words.

Finally, we are still a long way from a full understanding of the nature of the interaction between writing and reading. Simultaneous reading and writing is possible, which points to a degree of independence. Further, it is possible for the same patient to have qualitatively different acquired dyslexic and dysgraphic syndromes, and acquired "letter-by-letter" readers may identify words by a reverse employment of their spelling systems. Some of the more peripheral processes must be specialized for only writing or reading, but there is active current debate about how far "in" that specialization extends. In particular, there is disagreement about whether word production in writing and word recognition in reading are the responsibilities of one lexicon or two.

7 Learning to Read and Write

Young children typically begin to learn to read when they are about five years old. By that age the normal child can understand and use in speech several hundred words; that is, the child has many units in its auditory word recognition system and its phonemic word production system. Those systems will continue to develop in size as the child grows older but are already well established before reading and writing begin to be acquired. Also well established will be the grammatical processes responsible for comprehending and assembling spoken utterances (though, again, these will not yet have completed their development). So our novice reader and writer already possesses, albeit in incomplete form, many of the information-processing components which will be used in reading and writing. What he or she lacks are those processes which are *specific* to reading and writing—the processes of letter identification, visual word recognition, grapheme-phoneme conversion, graphemic word production, phoneme-grapheme conversion, letter execution, and the like. How these components are acquired, and how they are interlinked with the pre-existing speech processing components, are what cognitive psychologists interested in the acquisition of literacy must explain.

There has been an enormous amount of work done on learning to read and write, but little of it from the cognitive perspective adopted in this book. Nevertheless, interest in this area is growing and it is possible to tell a fairly consistent story from the work that has been done. We shall begin by considering how normal children learn to read.

MARSH, FRIEDMAN, WELCH, AND DESBERG'S
FOUR-STAGE THEORY OF LEARNING TO READ

Reading is not a biologically evolved skill like walking or talking. It is, rather, a product of cultural evolution and is dependent on cultural transmission for its continued existence. While one might accept the concept of a natural sequence of stages through which all children will pass in learning to walk or talk, there is no compelling reason to expect the same to be true of learning to read. That said, there is a sequence of stages which seems to capture quite well the way that many children in present-day Britain and America learn to read. That sequence has been described by Marsh, Friedman, Welch, and Desberg (1981).

Stage One: Glance-and-guess

As a first step in learning to read young children are often taught to recognize a smallish set of words by sight. This can be done using flash cards or simple stories. The child in this first stage is gradually establishing a set of visual letter and word recognition units. As yet the child has few or no phonic skills and so blocks at an unfamiliar word if it is encountered without any useful context. With such words the child is unable to produce any response. If, however, the same unfamiliar word is encountered in a sentence or story, then the child will often guess at a likely word using the previous context as a guide. For example, if the word *rocket* is not yet part of a child's sight vocabulary, then that child might read *The boy went to the moon in a rocket* as "The boy went to the moon in a spaceship," using the context to make a plausible guess at the last word.

During this first stage, a word guessed will often look nothing like the word on the page—all that matters is that the guess should fit the context. Because these guesses are adapted to the narrative of the story being read, Critchley and Critchley (1978) call them "narremic substitutions." Critchley and Critchley go on to draw a parallel between these errors and the semantic errors made by acquired deep dyslexics. This parallel is misguided, however, because of the different situations in which the errors occur. The child who reads *The boy went to the moon in a rocket* as "The boy went to the moon in a spaceship" does, in a sense, produce a semantic error by reading *rocket* as "spaceship" but (a) that child would never, as a deep dyslexic would, read the word *rocket* as "spaceship" when shown *rocket* in isolation, and (b) we could replace *rocket* by *cauliflower* in the above sentence and the child would just as readily assert that the boy travelled to the moon in a spaceship! We can easily be misled by the semantic relationship between *rocket* and *spaceship* into thinking that the child has extracted some meaning from *rocket* whereas, in actual fact, all that has happened is that the child has used the context to select a plausible word from out of his or her phonemic word production system.

Stage Two: Sophisticated guessing

Still within the first year of learning to read, the average child will progress into Stage Two of Marsh, Friedman, Welch, and Desberg's developmental sequence. The child still identifies words by sight alone, and is building up an ever larger set of visual word recognition units, but he or she is now more willing to respond to an unfamiliar word shown in isolation. The new word is typically named as one of the words the child *has* met in print before, and usually there is a degree of visual similarity between the written word and the response given. We have already met this strategy in Chapter 4—it is the strategy of "approximate visual access" used by acquired visual and phonological dyslexics. In another respect young children in Stages One and Two resemble acquired phonological dyslexics: they can happily read any word for which they have a visual word recognition unit, but their lack of phonic skills prevents them from being able to sound out and pronounce an unfamiliar word by applying grapheme-phoneme conversion processes.

When a Stage Two child runs into an unfamiliar word in a sentence or story, the context is once again used to constrain the guess. Where the Stage Two child differs from the Stage One child is that, once again, the guess is now drawn from only that set of words that the child has met in print before. Further, there is again some visual similarity now between the printed word and the response given. Biemiller (1970) likewise noted that errors made by beginning readers are usually appropriate to the context but may be visually quite unlike the target word. Soon, however, error words start to resemble the target word visually. Initially only the first letter is important, but by the end of the first year of reading Biemiller found that target and error words were beginning to share middle and end letters too.

To summarize, the child in Stage One is just beginning to read, and is gradually acquiring a set of visual word recognition units (his "sight vocabulary"). When a new word is encountered, the child will use the context to select from out of his phonemic word production system a likely word, making no use of the appearance of the new word. The child enters Stage Two when he starts to use context plus appearance of a new word to select as a guess a word that is within his growing visual word recognition system. The strategy used is the strategy of approximate visual access—looking for overlap between the visual characteristics of the new word and the stored specifications of the visual word recognition units. It is possible that the requirements of recognition units are at first only loosely specified anyway—perhaps the beginning and end letters, together with some indication of the overall length of the word. Approximate visual access can be used without context to guess at a new word in isolation, something the Stage One child cannot do.

Stage Three: The acquisition of simple grapheme-phoneme correspondences

The point soon arises when the child begins to be taught, or to see for himself or herself, that many letters or letter groups are pronounced the same in different words, and that one might therefore be able to work out what a new word is by sounding it out. The child, who is perhaps seven years old by now, is entering Marsh, Friedman, Welch, and Desberg's (1980) Stage Three. Initially this sounding out or "decoding" works in a simple left-to-right manner. For a time the decoding procedures tend not to be sensitive to the other letters surrounding the letter being pronounced. This means that a nonword like *cime* will be pronounced "kimmeh," first because the child is not yet aware of the context-sensitive rule that *c* is pronounced /s/ when it occurs before *i* at the beginning of a word (compare *city, cinema, circle*, etc.) and, second, because the child does not yet lengthen a vowel in response to a final *e* (compare *dim/dime, pin/pine, strip/stripe*, etc.).

Attempts at decoding new words are likely to result in some responses which are themselves nonwords (e.g., *choir* with a "ch," or *watch* pronounced so as to rhyme with "catch"). The occasional production of nonwords distinguishes the Stage Three child from Stage One and Two children, all of whose errors are real words.

Despite these limitations, the Stage Three child still becomes a far more versatile and independent reader because he or she now has a chance of being able to successfully decode a new word. Note that if a word occurs in context it may not be necessary to decode it all before it can be identified. Even many irregular words will yield to intelligent decoding. *Castle*, for instance, is an irregular word, but in most of its natural contexts decoding the regular initial portion *cas* will be sufficient to permit fairly sure identification. At the same time it should be emphasized that decoding will always remain just an option. *Castle* will soon come to join the expanding set of familiar words identified visually. What the acquisition of phonic skills does is to add a second, and valuable strategy for coping with alphabetic writing.

Stage Four: The skilled reader

The decoding skills of the Stage Three reader are still fairly basic, but as the child grows older they become more sophisticated. In Stage Four rules become context-sensitive so that *c* is pronounced /s/ before *i*, but /k/ before *o*, and vowels are lengthened by a final *e*. In addition, according to Marsh and his colleagues, the Stage Four child begins to use *analogy* as an alternative device for decoding. We have seen evidence in Chapter 3 that adults may use analogies to pronounce nonwords (recall the experiments of Glushko, 1979, and Kay and Marcel, 1981). Marsh *et al.* state that whereas a Stage Three child will decode *faugh* as "faw" and *tepherd* as "tefferd" through the application of rules, the Stage Four child at least on some occasions read *faugh* as "faff" by analogy with *laugh*, and *tepherd* as "tep-herd" by analogy with *shepherd*.

Stage Four is, in fact, the highest stage in the acquisition of literacy— the stage of adult-type skilled reading which we sought to describe and at least partially explain in Chapters 2, 3, and 5. One may continue to improve on the efficiency and scope of one's reading processes after one enters Stage Four somewhere between the ages of eight and ten, but the nature of the total system does not undergo any further qualitative changes.

Having described what seems to be the common developmental sequence we shall now discuss some aspects of it and variations on it. First, we shall briefly discuss the similarity between Stage Three and Four readers and acquired surface dyslexics. Second we shall consider how children use context when reading and, third, we shall look at the teaching of reading and how different teaching methods influence the acquisition of different reading strategies.

SIMILARITIES BETWEEN YOUNG READERS AND ACQUIRED SURFACE DYSLEXICS

Surface dyslexics, it will be recalled, are adults who, as a result of brain injury, have lost much of their former ability to identify words by sight. As a consequence they must attempt to decode most words phonically. This means that they can read regular words more successfully than irregular words, that a proportion of their errors are nonwords, and that they comprehend words as they pronounce them (e.g., *listen* "liston . . . the boxer"). All of these characteristics are also true of young (and not so young) readers in Stages Three and Four of Marsh, Friedman, Welch, and Desberg's developmental sequence.

Let us begin with the comparison between regular and irregular words. Jayne Simpson (1983) asked normal nine-year-old children to read aloud thirty-nine regular and thirty-nine irregular words taken from Coltheart, Besner, Jonasson, and Davelaar (1979). Twenty-one children were tested individually, and each was asked simply to read aloud the words which were printed on cards and shown one at a time. The children read correctly, on average, eighty-nine percent of the regular words, but seventy-two percent of the irregular words. Each child will have been familiar with some of the words shown. When a word is familiar it will be identified by its visual word recognition unit and pronounced via its phonemic word production unit, and the question of whether it is alphabetically regular or irregular is irrelevant. Give that the regular and irregular words were matched on frequency of occurrence in written English, then a roughly equal proportion of regular and irregular words should have been named using this "direct" route.

To see how the regular words gained their advantage we must look at the errors the children made. Fifty-four percent of the errors were nonwords. These were quite clearly unsuccessful attempts at phonic decoding (e.g., *thorough* read as "thorruff," *gauge* as "gugg,"and *yacht* as "yatsht"). These are decoding errors, and they are very like the errors of acquired surface dyslexics, but the decoding strategy must have worked on many occasions, particularly when applied to regular words. Some of the unfamiliar irregular words like *flood* or *prove* might also have been guessed correctly on the basis of phonic decoding, particularly if the child was a Stage Four child capable of using analogies. Nevertheless, decoding will undoubtedly be successful more often when applied to regular words than to irregular words, and this is where the differences arise. It is worth making the more general point that in this case as in others, analyzing the errors is not a failsafe guide to how correct responses come about: although many of the errors made by the nine-year-olds were phonic, many of their *correct* responses must have occurred as a result of direct, visual recognition.

Not all of the children's errors were nonwords, and there was an interesting difference between the regular and irregular words in the extent to which they induced real word or nonword errors. Sixty-one percent of the errors to irregular words were nonwords whereas only twenty-nine percent of the errors to regular words were nonwords. A possible explanation for this finding is that although these nine-year-olds have developed some phonic skills they may not have entirely abandoned the strategy of visual approximation—looking for visual overlap between a new letter string and the requirements of an existing visual word recognition unit. As a broad generalization, irregular words tend to be visually distinctive and are therefore less likely than regular words to overlap sufficiently with the specifications of an existing recognition unit to cause it to form the basis of a response based on visual approximation. Irregular words will tend, therefore, to be subjected to the alternative strategy of phonic recoding more than will the regular words. Since visual approximation yields real word errors while phonic recoding yields a proportion of nonword errors, we can see why irregular words should induce a higher proportion of nonword errors than regular words.

Acquired surface dyslexics comprehend words as they pronounce them, and so do normal children. Simpson (1983) asked a group of nine-year-olds to define each word they were shown before naming it and obtained many errors like *mown* read as 'in the sky . . . moon," *lever* as "meat you eat . . . liver," or *dough* as "a bird . . . dove."

The parallel between young readers and surface dyslexics has been drawn before by Marcel (1980) and by Coltheart, Masterson, Byng, Prior, and Critchlow (1983), but it is perhaps worth repeating that the comparison applies only to Stage Three and Four readers. Stage One and Two readers resemble phonological rather than surface dyslexics. The reason Stage Three and Four readers resemble surface dyslexics is not hard to see. Surface dyslexics have lost access to many of the units in their visual word recognition system and so are obliged to rely heavily on phonic mediation. Young readers have not yet *established* visual word recognition units for many words they will eventually be able to recognize by sight, and so must also depend to a considerable extent on phonic decoding when trying to name unfamiliar words and phonic mediation when trying to understand them.

CHILDREN'S USE OF CONTEXT IN READING

We have already commented on the tendency of children to use the context in which a word occurs to constrain their guess as to what it might be. The resulting errors, called "narremic substitutions" earlier in this chapter, are generally words which fit the preceding context both grammatically and semantically (cf. Weber, 1968). Goodman (1967) has cited these errors in support of his belief that, "reading is a psycholinguistic guessing game . . . [which] does not result from precise perception and identification of all elements, but from skill in selecting the fewest, most productive cues necessary to produce guesses which are right the first time" (p. 127). Goodman believes that skilled readers make heavy use of context to actively anticipate forthcoming words, and that only enough visual analysis is done to confirm or disconfirm these predictions. He argues that narremic substitutions signal a child who is reading in an intelligent, adultlike way, and he urges teachers to deal leniently with the child who commits such errors.

Although Goodman's view has been influential, and probably harmless as educational theories go, it may be based on an incorrect view of the nature of skilled reading. First of all, because children use preceding context to generate a guess when faced with an unfamiliar word does not mean that they always use context to aid identification of familiar words. Further, as was pointed out in Chapter 5, the computational effort required to continually enumerate sets of likely words would be enormous and cannot be regarded as in any way simpler or more natural than allowing the stimulus information to guide identification. We have seen in Chapter 5 that skilled readers probably make extensive use of context only when the stimulus quality is poor, though less skilled readers appear to make more use of context. Children seem to be like less skilled older readers in this respect (Ehrlich, 1981; Perfetti and Roth, 1981). For example, West and Stanovich (1978) required nine-year-olds, eleven-year-olds, and adults to name words presented either in isolation or after incomplete sentence contexts. The nine- and eleven-year-olds were faster at naming the words shown in contexts than those in isolation but the adults showed no difference; they did not seem to use the incomplete sentences to predict the word to be named or prime the recognition units for likely completion words.

Even children may vary in their use of context depending on how skilled they are as readers. Perfetti, Goldman, and Hogoboam (1979) found that skilled eight- to ten-year-old readers made less use of sentence contexts to facilitate word naming speed than did unskilled readers of the same age. This implies that even by the age of eight or ten children's stimulus-driven identification processes may be becoming so efficient that the immature reliance on context is already disappearing.

THE INFLUENCE OF TEACHING METHODS ON THE ACQUISITION OF READING STRATEGIES

While the developmental sequence described by Marsh, Friedman, Welch, and Desberg (1980) may be a natural one, there is no reason to believe it to be a necessary sequence. Surely no one could deny that one could, in principle, teach children a range of correspondences between letters or letter groups and sounds, before introducing the first word. For example, if one first taught a child the normal sound values of *g*, *d*, and *o*, and only then showed the child the word *dog*, the child's first access to meaning from print would be via phonic recoding and the auditory word recognition system. That said, after two or three such readings, there is no reason to believe that the child would not establish a visual word recognition unit for *dog*, and thereafter recognize it entirely visually.

The sort of teaching method just described is, of course, an extreme case of a "phonic" regime. Phonic teaching has traditionally been contrasted with "whole-word" or "look-and-say" methods which are aimed at encouraging recognition of words by sight (see Chall, 1967, for an account of the historical debate between these two approaches). Attempts have been made to compare the effectiveness of these two methods, but there are several problems, one of which is that there is no such thing as a pure phonics or pure look-and-say reading scheme; schemes simply differ in the relative emphasis they place upon phonic skills and the development of a sight vocabulary. A second problem is that most of the studies have used some fairly gross measure of reading achievement. They have tended not to provide information on such things as the types of errors made by children; information which can be revealing as to the reading strategies being used by them.

An exception to this generalization is the study by Barr (1974) who begins by summarizing some previous research showing that children taught by look-and-say tend to make errors that are real words and are drawn from the set of words they have met in print before (like the Stage Two children discussed earlier). In contrast, children taught by more phonic methods will produce some nonwords when trying to decode words, and will draw their real word errors from their entire spoken vocabulary. Barr was interested in the extent to which teaching methods determine children's preferred reading strategies and examined the reading performance of a group of thirty-two five- to six-year-olds in December and May of their first year at school (that is, after about three and eight months of instruction). Half the children were taught by look-and-say methods which stressed visual recognition without breaking words down into letters and sounds. The remaining half of the children were taught by phonic methods, and so learned how to sound out the letters in a word and blend them together.

Barr classified individual children as "phonic" or "sight-word" readers independently of the teaching group they were in. Phonic readers made occasional nonword errors and drew their errors from a large vocabulary. Sight-word readers produced no nonwords and drew their errors from the smaller set of words already met in print. By December of the first year Barr found that ten of the sixteen children taught by phonic methods were in fact phonic readers. The remaining six were sight-word readers who seemed not to have benefited from the phonic training, but had apparently learned to recognize by sight the real words used to illustrate the phonic sounds of letters. By May of the first year, however, five of these six children were now phonic readers and only one of the group of sixteen children receiving phonic instruction remained a resolute sight-word reader.

Turning to the group who were receiving look-and-say instruction, by December of their first year fifteen were sight-word readers but one was a phonic reader. Perhaps this child was being given covert phonic training at home, or perhaps he or she just was an individual to whom phonics came more naturally than whole-word visual word recognition. By May that child had, however, succumbed and become a sight-word reader, but another child—the best reader in the group—had begun to develop phonic skills of its own accord. Again, we cannot be certain about the effects of home influences, but it is possible that some children taught by look-and-say will begin to make their own phonic inferences based on the more regular correspondences they encounter.

So, the nature of the teaching method used had a strong influence on the development of children's reading strategies, though sometimes this clashed with the child's preferred and natural strategy. One of the whole-word group started to develop phonic skills of the child's own accord, and it would have been interesting to see if more would have in time, though even if they did that is no reason for not teaching phonics explicitly at some stage. As has been noted earlier, if real words are used to exemplify letter-sound correspondences, then so-called "phonic" teaching will also tutor direct, visual word recognition as children become familiar with words and establish recognition units for them.

We shall have a little more to say about teaching at the end of this chapter, but first we shall examine how children learn to write and, in particular, how they learn to spell.

LEARNING TO WRITE

The child who is starting to learn how to write faces a number of hurdles. First, he or she must master the style of language used in writing. Much of the language we use in everyday life occurs in conversational give-and-take, and is in a style different from that we use when writing (Olson, 1977). However, as was noted in Chapter 5, we approach the normal writing style in speech when we tell a story or relate the events of the day in an uninterrupted monologue. Encouraging young children to use this explicit style of speech with well-formed sentences should make the transition to the writing style less abrupt.

Writing is a motor act as well as a linguistic one, and a second problem for the child is learning how to form letters and orient them on the page. While such things as letter confusions (between *b* and *d*, for example, or *m* and *w*), fusions of adjacent letters, and reverse "mirror writing" of words may give cause for concern in an older child, they are exceedingly common in young children who are still trying to acquire the perceptual-motor coordination required for fluent writing.

There has been some research done into children's acquisition of the written style of language (Frederiksen and Dominic, 1982; Kress, 1982), and some too into the motoric aspects of learning to write (Søvik, 1975; Thomassen and Teulings, 1979), but most of the research on learning to write has focused on a third source of difficulty—learning how to spell. For better or for worse, our society places great emphasis on being able to spell correctly. An application for a job is unlikely to be successful if it is replete with misspellings. Perhaps this is why learning to spell has attracted the attention it has over the years.

How do children learn to spell?

If psychologists and others have been quick to believe (wrongly) that young children read predominantly or exclusively via sound, they have been even quicker to believe that children habitually spell via sound. While it is easy to see how this belief has arisen, the truth is, as always, more complex than such simple generalizations can capture. A child who knows the common correspondences between sounds and letters can attempt to assemble a candidate spelling for a word based on the way it is pronounced. If the word is a regular one, then the assembled spelling has a chance of being correct. However, we saw in Chapter 6 that because a word is regular as far as spelling-to-sound correspondence is concerned does not mean that its spelling is necessarily going to be predictable from its pronunciation. *Lame, croak,* and *weed* are regular words in that they are pronounced as one would expect from their spellings, but if one knew only their pronunciations then one could equally well assemble *LAIM, CROKE,* and *WEDE* as candidate spellings. This means that phonically mediated spelling must be a highly error-prone process for anyone, whether child or adult, to employ as a primary spelling strategy. Any child who reliably spells "cat" as *cat* and never as *KAT,* or "mummy" as *mummy* and never as *MUMI* must be retrieving the spellings of *cat* and *mummy* from his or her graphemic word production system, even if that system only contains half a dozen words.

Another point worth making is that words are only regular by reference to their pronunciation in a particular dialect, usually the dominant, "educated" dialect. A word which is regular for a speaker of this dialect may be irregular for a child who speaks in a regional or ethnic dialect or accent. Orton (1931) gives examples of assembled phonic misspellings based on the pronunciation of words by children from Boston, Massachusetts (for example, *INVERTATION* for *invitation, DANGERSS* for *dangerous, GARROWSCOPE* for *gyroscope,* and *SPECALATIN* for *speculating*). Desberg, Elliott, and Marsh (1980) note that the pronunciations of many words in Black American English makes their spellings unpredictable by phonic assembly. While this means that a natural strategy—that of phonic assembly—is less useful to speakers of supposedly "nonstandard" dialects, the end point of development, where the spellings of all familiar words are retrieved as wholes from the graphemic word production system, will be the same for all literate adults.

The nature of the English spelling system dictates that reliable spelling must be done by retrieving spellings from a word production system rather than assembling them from their sounds. That said, there is some evidence to suggest that children may develop the strategy of phonically mediated spelling earlier and perhaps more spontaneously than they develop phonically mediated reading. Read (1971) and C. Chomsky (1970) describe preschool children who have spontaneously created their own spelling systems and spell words as they pronounce them. Read and Chomsky show how these children's spellings can yield insights into their systems of sound representation, segmentation, and categorization.

Bryant and Bradley (1980) gave some normal six- and seven-year-olds a list of thirty words to read on one occasion and to write on another. They found that being able to read a word was no guarantee of being able to spell it, and vice-versa. The four words most commonly read correctly but misspelled were *school, light, train,* and *egg*. These are all visually rather distinctive words which cannot reliably be spelled phonically (compare *SKULE, LITE, TRANE,* and *EG*). In contrast, the four words most commonly spelled correctly but read incorrectly were the visually nondescript words *bun, pat, leg,* and *mat* whose spellings nevertheless have a fair chance of being successfully predicted from their sounds. Interestingly many of the same six- and seven-year-olds later succeeded in reading *bun, pat, leg,* and *mat* correctly when those words were embedded in a list of nonwords which obliged the children to adopt a phonic reading strategy.

Bryant and Bradley's children seem to have preferred to read visually, though they could switch to assembling pronunciations phonically when forced. They often failed, however, to make this switch spontaneously. In terms of Marsh, Friedman, Welch, and Desberg's (1981) scheme they were probably at the transition from Stage Two to Stage Three. When it came to spelling, they must have spelled some words as wholes, but were much more ready in this case to use phonic assembly as a strategy. This conclusion is reinforced by Bryant and Bradley's (1980) finding that five-year-old children's spelling errors tend to be more "phonic" than their reading errors.

It is the fact that children are so quick to spell "cough" as *KOFF* and "laugh" as *LAFF* that has made psychologists so ready to accept a phonic mediation account of all children's spelling. Here again we see the dangers inherent in extrapolating incautiously from what happens when errors are produced to what happens when correct responses are produced. Errors can be highly informative, but like all forms of data they must be interpreted with care. Learning to spell a word does not mean learning how to reliably assemble its spelling from its sound, rather it means establishing a graphemic word production unit and being able to access that unit when required.

Some children may be more reliant than others on retrieving spellings from their graphemic word production systems. Dodd (1980) found that profoundly deaf children make a far smaller proportion of "phonetic" spelling errors than hearing children, suggesting that deaf children, as one might expect, are poor at phonically mediated spelling and rely on storing spellings in, and retrieving spellings from, a graphemic word production system. As a consequence, deaf children do not show the superior spellings of regular words over irregular words that hearing children show. Another group of children who seem to spell largely "by rote" (i.e., by retrieval from the graphemic word production system) are children with developmental pronunciation difficulties—children who pronounce "train" as "tain," "ship" as "tip," or "pin" as "bin." These children spell irregular words as well as they spell regular words and, in a manner reminiscent of patient R. D. (see pp. 70-71), their ability to spell a word is independent of whether they can pronounce it correctly or not. Thus they may be able to spell *train* and *ship* correctly while pronouncing them "tain" and "tip" (Robinson, Beresford, and Dodd, 1982).

Young spellers and surface dysgraphics

Just as young children at Stages Three and Four resemble acquired surface dyslexics in their reading, so they resemble acquired surface dysgraphics in their spelling. Surface dysgraphics, it will be recalled, have lost access to many of the words in their graphemic word production systems, and so must resort to spelling phonically many words they would hitherto have retrieved as wholes. Because of this bias to the phonic route they are more successful at spelling regular words to dictation than irregular words, and their errors are predominantly phonic.

Precisely the same pattern is found in young children who, rather than having lost access to many graphemic word production units, have yet to acquire them. Hatfield and Patterson (1983) note the close similarity between the errors of their surface dysgraphic patient T. P. (discussed in Chapter 5) and those of a normal eight-year-old girl of their acquaintance, and Barron (1980) and Seymour and Porpodas (1980) have observed superior spelling to dictation of regular than irregular words by seven- to twelve-year-olds.

In Chapter 5 we also mentioned the tendency of T. P. to substitute real word homophones as errors. Homophone spelling errors have been reported in normal children by Plessas (1963) and Doctor (1978). Doctor asked six- to ten-year-olds to write down dictated sentences. The sentences contained homophones like "sew," "knew," "wood," or "no," but the context in which the homophone was heard made it clear which meaning was implied. Despite this the children made many homophone errors. For example, sixty percent of the times "sew" was misspelt by six-year-olds it was as *SO* or *SOW* (other errors included *SOE, SOWE, ZOE*, etc.). These errors occurred even if the erroneous version of the homophone was itself irregular; thus "wood" was frequently misspelled as *WOULD*, and "no" as *KNOW*. These errors imply that the graphemic word production system could be involved in phonic spelling when word-sized units can be found embedded in a longer, unfamiliar word. Examples of this taken from Orton (1931) include children misspelling "taxation" as *TACKSAYTION*, "thievish" as *THEVEFISH*, and "frequently" as *FREAKWENTLY*. The principle of using the largest available unit to translate from one language code to another (in this case from sound to print) which was discussed in earlier chapters may apply to children's spelling too.

TEACHING READING AND WRITING

The age at which children receive their first formal reading instruction varies somewhat from country to country, ranging from around five years in countries such as Great Britain, India, and Uruguay, through six in the United States, France, and Japan, to seven in Denmark and Sweden (figures from Downing, 1973). Between the 1930s and 1960s it was not uncommon to encounter the claim being made that normal children needed to achieve a state of "reading readiness" before they could be successfully taught to read, and that this state was usually reached at around the age of six and a half. Coltheart (1979) has shown that the early studies on which this claim was based simply could not bear the weight of the conclusions placed upon them, either because they were methodologically flawed or because they just did not find what they were commonly said to have found. Certainly many children with a mental age of less than six and a half make substantial progress in learning to read, though Coltheart (1979) reviews several studies showing that effort put into teaching children to read at a very early age has few, if any, long-term benefits because the late starters soon catch up with the early achievers once they have begun to receive instruction.

To a cognitive psychologist the concept of reading readiness does not come naturally. In 1925 a group of 560 American teachers of first grade (five- or six-year-old) children were asked what, in their opinion, constituted "reading readiness." Their replies included appropriate comprehension, sufficient command of English, good speaking vocabulary, and wide and varied experiences (Holmes, 1928). These teachers knew what cognitive psychologists now assert, namely that reading draws on a number of psychological processes and skills, many of which are not specific to reading, and many of which begin their development well before children start to read.

In Chapter 5 it was argued that the comprehension of written sentences and longer texts draws on processes which are also used to understand spoken language, though the style used in writing tends to be rather different from the style used in conversational give and take. We also saw in Chapter 5 how knowledge of the world is directly utilized in sentence comprehension (remember the city council versus the protestors). Obviously the young child with a wide general knowledge who is used to being read to and listening to stories is going to have a headstart when it comes to reading stories and texts over the child with a restricted knowledge base who is only used to the conversational style of language. Similarly, writing involves the skill of composing text made up of well-formed, well-connected, and explicit sentences. Children can begin to master this style in speech before they begin writing by being encouraged to relate stories, or describe episodes in their day to others who were not present at the event so must be provided with all the necessary details.

Reading and writing both draw in concrete, information-processing terms on a child's aural vocabulary. A child for whom many words being met in his reading books are utterly unfamiliar has to create a new visual word recognition unit, learn a new meaning, and establish a new phonemic word production unit for each new word. In contrast, the child with a larger speech vocabulary will have the word meanings and phonemic production units already present and has the lesser task of just connecting a new visual word recognition unit up to those pre-existing components. Likewise, a child may have acquired some skill at decoding unfamiliar words to sounds, but that child will be unable to complete the phonically mediated access to meaning unless the child has *heard* the word before, because phonic access to meaning relies on an internally generated acoustic form being able to trigger an already existing auditory word recognition unit. Thus, the phonic skills acquired in Stage Three and Four of learning to read will be of reduced value if a child does not have the necessary spoken vocabulary because, as we illustrated earlier in the book with the *phoks* and *yott* examples, the point of having an alphabet is that it enables you to identify a word which is already part of your auditory vocabulary when you encounter it for the first time in print.

Linguistic awareness

When we speak, our words are formed from strings of the distinctive sounds which we call phonemes. This is true whether we are literate or illiterate. At the same time many children, and indeed some adults, find it hard to divide a spoken word up into its component phonemes if asked to list or count them. Psychologists who have studied this skill refer to it as an aspect of "linguistic awareness"; the conscious understanding and manipulation of the units of one's spoken language (see Liberman, Liberman, Mattingly, and Shankweiler, 1980, and Rozin and Gleitman, 1977, for reviews).

It has been shown several times that good readers are better at phonemic segmentation than poor readers, but the correct interpretation of this finding is unclear (Golinkoff, 1978). Is it that good linguistic awareness assists the acquisition of literacy, or is it that learning to read and write improves children's awareness of words as sequences of sounds? Morais, Cary, Alegria, and Bertelson (1979) carried out a study in Portugal comparing the segmentation abilities of literate adults with those of other adults who, purely because of the circumstances in which they had grown up, had never learned to read or write. The illiterate adults possessed some capacity for phonemic segmentation but were much less good than their literate counterparts. This suggests that learning to read and write to some extent makes one more aware of the nature of language as a medium.

The teaching method used also appears to play a part here. Alegria, Pignot, and Morais (1982) found that children taught by phonic methods were better than children taught by whole-word methods at reversing the phonemes of a one-syllable, two-phoneme word or nonword (e.g., saying "lo" given "ol"). This is presumably because phonic methods draw more attention to the sounds of language than do whole-word methods.

Though learning to read and write probably heightens awareness of the sounds of one's language, there is also evidence that children who come to reading with good linguistic awareness fare better than those less conscious of their language as an object in itself rather than a means to a communicative end. Bradley and Bryant (1983) assessed the linguistic awareness of 403 four- and five-year-olds, none of whom had any measurable ability to read or spell. This was done by giving the children three or four three-letter words, all but one of which had the same initial, middle, or final sound. The child's task was to say which word was the "odd man out." For example, if the experimenter said "lot, cot, hat, pot" then the child had to identify "hat" as the odd man out. Similarly, if the list were "pin, win, sit, fin", then "sit" is the odd man out.

Bradley and Bryant found that a child's performance in this task before any reading or writing had begun was an important predictor of how well he or she would have learned to read and write three or four years later.

In addition to this, Bradley and Bryant (1983) looked at the effects on learning to read and write of training children in phonemic awareness. A group of children with poor language awareness were trained in forty sessions spread over two years at selecting which of a set of pictures of common objects had names with the same beginning (e.g., hen, hat), middle (e.g., hen, pet) or final (e.g., hen, man) sounds. At the end of the training these children were reading and spelling better than a group given no special training. Training children to classify pictures into categories such as "farm animals" had no effect, but a group taught to classify by sounds, and then taught which letters represented these sounds, fared even better in learning to read and write. None of the training schedules had any effect on childrens' arithmetic skills.

Bradley and Bryant's study provides the first clear evidence that making young children aware of the sounds of their language will help them learn to read and write. If there is a criticism to be made of this study, it is perhaps that reading and spelling were only assessed by a standard reading and spelling test. A question which has not been posed as often as it might have been by researchers into linguistic awareness and reading is the question of what *aspects* of the acquisition of literacy require the awareness and manipulation of individual language sounds. Whole-word visual identification and naming of familiar words does not; neither does whole-word retrieval and production of spelling. Where phoneme segmentation and manipulation may play a part is in phonic decoding of unfamiliar words and phonic assembly of spellings. For example, one would predict that, when all other factors are controlled, "linguistic awareness" might not be relevant to children's reading performance in Stages One and Two, but it might affect the age of transition into Stage Three. Also, the capacity to spell phonically may be more affected by language awareness than the capacity for the storage and reproduction of learned spellings.

That said, training language awareness clearly does help children develop at least some of the component skills which literacy draws upon. In addition to the sort of training used in Bradley and Bryant's study, language awareness can be developed by rhyming games, "I spy," by looking for objects beginning with the same sound, and so on. Bradley's (1980) *Assessing Reading Difficulties: A diagnostic and remedial approach* contains much sensible and practical advice on the teaching of reading and writing, not just to poor readers, and suggests that time spent in the home, nursery school, or kindergarten on developing awareness of language sounds would be wisely invested.

Finally, let us not forget that if adults read at all they do so for information and enjoyment. Downing and Leong (1982) review evidence that children retain more and progress better if they find the books they are given to read interesting. There can be no substitute for enjoyment.

SUMMARY OF CHAPTER 7

Learning to read and write requires the integration of new skills specific to processing written language with existing skills already developed for the comprehension and production of speech. Marsh, Friedman, Welch, and Desberg (1981) have outlined a developmental sequence which describes how many children learn to read. In Stage One words are identified as wholes through the acquisition of visual word recognition units. The child lacks any phonic skills. Unfamiliar words out of context elicit no response. Unfamiliar words in context may elicit a guess based on the preceding context which bears no visual resemblance to the word on the page. In Stage Two recognition is still visual without any phonics, but guesses now come to be drawn from within the set of words the child has encountered in print before, and the guesses bear an increasing visual resemblance to the target. In Stage Three the child begins to acquire simple letter-to-sound correspondences so may now attempt to decode or "sound out" a new word. In Stage Four the use of phonics becomes more advanced and may incorporate the use of analogies as well as correspondences.

In Stages One and Two young readers resemble acquired phonological dyslexics while in Stages Three and Four they resemble acquired surface dyslexics (because the number of words for which they possess visual recognition units is still limited so they must frequently resort to phonic decoding and phonically mediated access to meaning). The strategy of approximate visual access appears to persist alongside phonic decoding in young Stage Three and Four readers. It is not clear when, if ever, it ceases to be employed. Throughout their development children use context to aid their attempts at word identification, though reliance on context is probably the hallmark of an immature or poor reader, something which declines as reading skill increases.

Teaching methods can undoubtedly influence the rate at which children progress through the different stages. Indeed, children taught by strongly phonic methods may never show some of the Stage One and Two characteristics, though words decoded phonically on the first few encounters will soon come to be recognized visually as wholes.

Learning to write involves mastering that language style most commonly encountered in written English, learning the spellings of words, and learning the art of letter and word formation. Words spelled reliably and correctly must be spelled from memory (i.e., from the graphemic word production system) though children seem to take to phonic spelling much earlier and much more naturally than they take to phonic reading. Once again, the fact that childrens' graphemic production systems are limited, so that they must rely on phonic assembly when asked to spell many words, means that their spelling resembles that of acquired surface dysgraphics.

Because reading and writing share some processes in common with listening and speaking, developing those processes in the preliterate child will help in the later acquisition of literacy. Children use speech to communicate, and may not think about the nature and organization of what is for them a means to an end. Some children may only be made fully aware of language as a sequence of separable, distinctive sounds when they are taught to read or spell. At the same time, there is evidence that making very young children aware of the sounds of language (e.g., by rhyming and other word games) facilitates the later acquisition of reading and writing skills. There is also evidence that if children find their early encounters with print enjoyable they will progress better.

8 Developmental Dyslexia and Dysgraphia

THE CONCEPT OF DEVELOPMENTAL DYSLEXIA

In Chapter Four we discussed at length some of the many published reports of adults who were once skilled readers but who later found themselves experiencing reading difficulties as a consequence of brain injury such as a stroke. In some of these cases the problem is almost exclusively a reading difficulty, but in many cases other language functions are also impaired. No one seems to object to calling these patients "acquired dyslexics," or to the suggestion that acquired dyslexia comes in several different varieties. In contrast, the very concept of *developmental* dyslexia has sometimes been opposed, and the notion of *varieties* of developmental dyslexia has certainly not achieved universal acceptance.

What do psychologists have in mind when they say that a child is "dyslexic"? The definition of dyslexia proferred by the World Federation of Neurology is a follows:

> [Dyslexia is] a disorder manifested by difficulty in learning to read despite conventional instruction, adequate intelligence, and sociocultural opportunity. It is dependent upon fundamental cognitive disabilities which are frequently of constitutional origin. (Critchley, 1975)

There are a couple of points in this definition worth developing in a little more detail.

1. *Developmental dyslexics must have adequate intelligence.* This requirement is introduced in order to distinguish dyslexic children from children whose reading is poor for their age because they are *generally*

105

backward. That is, psychologists who use the term "dyslexia" usually wish to reserve if for children whose reading (and spelling) are *unexpectedly* and *discrepantly* poor. In practice this often means that a child must attain a certain standard of performance on an intelligence test (e.g., an IQ of ninety or more) in order to be considered as a candidate for the label "dyslexic."

2. *Developmental dyslexics must have experienced adequate reading instruction and sociocultural opportunity.* Obviously a bright child may fail to learn to read because he or she comes from a deprived background or has received inadequate teaching. One would not, however, necessarily want to call that child "dyslexic." Of course, such a child *could* be dyslexic, but it is impossible to rule out alternative explanations. Only if the background and schooling were improved and the child *still* failed to learn to read might one consider calling him or her dyslexic. Note, however, that requirements (1) and (2) mean that children diagnosed as dyslexic tend to be the bright offspring of "good" homes attending "good" schools. There is no reason to suppose that dyslexia is in any real sense a "middle-class disease," only that those tend to be the children where psychologists feel most confident they can exclude other obvious causes of reading failure.

IS DYSLEXIA A DISEASE?

Although the World Federation of Neurology definition of dyslexia claims that it is "frequently of constitutional origin," in practice the defining criteria are psychological and social. This means that questions like "How common is dyslexia?" have to be answered with care. To qualify as dyslexic a child's IQ must be of a certain level, his reading ability must be below what one would expect given his age and IQ, and his home and school must pass certain minimum requirements. Forgetting for a moment the issue of home and school standards, we might choose to call a child dyslexic if his IQ is, say, ninety or above (one hundred being average) and if his reading age as assessed by a standardized reading test is at least eighteen months below his actual chronological age. A survey of the school population using these criteria would uncover a certain percentage of children who qualified as dyslexic (perhaps around two to four percent). However, if we required an IQ of 110 or above and a reading age of, say, twenty-four months below actual age, then the percentage of apparently "dyslexic" children would decrease dramatically.

At this point the reader might feel tempted to say that if the number of "dyslexic" children in the population can be raised or lowered more or less at whim, then the very notion of dyslexia must be of dubious value. If dyslexia cannot be diagnosed like measles can be diagnosed, then perhaps it is not a very useful or sound concept. It is true that dyslexia is not a disease like measles, but that does not prevent the term from being useful psychologically or even medically. Consider, for instance, the concept of "obesity." A person is called "obese" if his or her weight substantially exceeds that of a normal person of the same height and sex. Much medical research has been done on obesity and progress has been made in understanding its causes. Nevertheless, the dividing line between "normal" and "obese" is entirely arbitrary and, as with dyslexia, one can raise or lower the percentage of people who are classed as obese simply by altering the criteria. Realizing this fact does not invalidate the concept of obesity (or the many other comparable medical terms) any more than it invalidates the concept of dyslexia.

Having said all that, there will undoubtedly be people reading this book who dislike the term "dyslexia" as applied to children. I am quite happy for them to use an alternative such as "specific reading retardation," "learning disability," or any of the many other equivalent terms in use— all that concerns me is that we should agree that there *are* intelligent children with reasonable backgrounds and educational opportunities who are nevertheless unexpectedly poor at reading and writing. If we can agree on that, then we can at least consider the viability of cognitive descriptions and explanations of the difficulties such children experience.

UNITARY EXPLANATIONS OF DEVELOPMENTAL DYSLEXIA

In the 1880s and 1890s much valuable work on acquired reading disorders was being done. The idea that there may be a developmental equivalent to the acquired dyslexias seems to have occurred independently to two British doctors named James Kerr and Pringle Morgan, both of whom presented their ideas publicly in 1896. Neither seems to have developed the notion further, but the idea was taken up by a Scottish ophthalmologist called James Hinshelwood whose work is summarized in his book of 1917 entitled *Congenital Word-Blindness*. In America the concept of developmental dyslexia was promoted by one Samuel T. Orton whose *Reading, Writing and Speech Problems in Children*, published in 1937, was highly influential. Over the years dyslexia research has been something of an industry and thousands of papers have been written on the subject. Access to this body of work may be gained through Vellutino's (1979) comprehensive book, and also through chapters in the book edited by Benton and Pearl (1978), Frith (1980b), Kavanagh and Venezky (1980), Pavlidis and Miles (1981), Pirozzolo and Wittrock (1981), Brainerd and Plessey (1982), and Malatesha and Aaron (1982).

To review all that work would be a monumental task of doubtful cost-effectiveness. One problem with a lot of dyslexia research is that investigators have often been determined to prove (a) that all developmental dyslexics are alike in their symptoms and difficulties, (b) that if developmental dyslexia is a unitary syndrome then it must have a single cause, and (c) that their particular theory explains the one and only cause and variety of dyslexia. Because these unitary explanations have exercised such a powerful grip over thinking about developmental dyslexia we shall briefly review some examples and discuss their shortcomings. In so doing we shall make some general methodological points about the proper conduct of studies which compare groups of normal and dyslexic subjects. We shall then go on to present evidence for the existence of *varieties* of developmental dyslexia with the attendant assumption of *multiple* cognitive causes.

Unitary hypothesis 1: "Dyslexia is a perceptual disorder"

It would be very difficult to learn to read if one was unable to extract visual information from the printed page, analyze the patterns in it, and retain those patterns (e.g., the forms of letters or words) for future reference. From time to time it has been proposed that developmental dyslexia is caused by some sort of general perceptual deficit, the details of which vary from theory to theory. These need not concern us, however, because there is now ample evidence, summarized by Vellutino (1979; 1981) and Mitchell (1982), that this proposal is incorrect. For example, Mason and Katz (1976) required dyslexic and normal children to search for a target shape in a set of other unfamiliar shapes and found no difference in the search rate of the two groups. Similarly, N. Ellis and Miles (1978) found no difference in the speed with which normal and dyslexic children could judge whether pairs of letters were the same or different.

Certainly there are "visual" tasks where dyslexics fare worse than normal children, and these are often tasks where alphabetic materials are used. The problem here is one which recurs again and again where dyslexic and normal children are compared, and it is that the poorer performance of the dyslexics may be a *consequence* rather than a *cause* of their difficulties in learning to read. Whatever the origins of dyslexia, the simple fact of having successfully learned to read, with the resulting development and practice of perceptual and verbal abilities, is likely to render normal children superior to dyslexics on a whole host of tasks where letters, words, and sentences are used. One way to reduce this problem is not to compare dyslexics only with normal children of the same age (the conventional "chronological age controls,") but to also compare them with normal children whose reading abilities are similar to those of the dyslexics; that is, to compare them with *younger, normal children* matched on something like reading age. Alas, most of the studies testing the perceptual deficit hypothesis have lacked a group of reading age controls. Despite that, there is still no reason to accept the perceptual disorder hypothesis as a unitary account of developmental dyslexia.

Unitary hypothesis 2: "Dyslexia is caused by faulty eye movements"

If one had congenital difficulty controlling one's eye movements, then learning to read would obviously present enormous problems. Ciuffreda, Bahill, Kenyon, and Stark (1976) discuss a case of an individual with deficient eye movement control who, unsurprisingly, experienced great difficulty with reading. Further, it has been demonstrated many times that dyslexics tend to show shorter saccades, longer fixations, and more regressions than normal readers (Rayner, 1978; Pavlidis, 1981). It is, however, a long way from such demonstrations to the claim made by Pavlidis (1981) that erratic eye movements may be the unitary cause of developmental dyslexia.

In attempting to evaluate this claim one immediately runs into the "cause or consequence" problem. Are erratic eye movements the cause of dyslexia or a consequence of failure to learn to read (in the same way that my eye movements when scanning a page of Hebrew or Chinese would doubtless be erratic)? Several authors, on reviewing the evidence, have opted for the consequence position (e.g., Rayner, 1978; N. Ellis and Miles, 1981; Mitchell, 1982). Mitchell (1982) discusses an experiment by Stanley (1978) which found differences in eye movement patterns between good and poor readers in a reading task but not in a task where subjects had to locate the picture of an object within a scene. Both tasks required efficient scanning, but only in the reading task could the two groups be discriminated. Finally, it is possible for the scores of two groups to be "significantly different" despite overlap between them. Thus, the measured eye movements of a dyslexic group could be significantly worse than those of a normal group though some of the "dyslexic" group may be obtaining better scores than some of the "normal" group. It has not been demonstrated that all of a randomly selected group of dyslexics show worse eye movements than all of a group of normal controls as would be necessary to establish the unitary deficient eye movement hypothesis. Readers wishing to pursue the issue of whether faulty eye movement control lies at the root of developmental dyslexia are referred to the exchange between Pavlidis and Stanley, Smith, and Howell, in the *British Journal of Psychology* for 1983 (Pavlidis, 1983; Stanley, Smith, and Howell, 1983a, b).

Unitary hypothesis 3: "Dyslexia is a disorder of short-term memory"

When standardized intelligence tests are given to normal and dyslexic children a common finding is that the dyslexics tend to do badly on tests of "memory span"; for example, the number of digits which can be repeated correctly after a single hearing (e.g., Rugel, 1974). Could it be that dyslexia is in some way caused by this short-term memory deficit? There are a number of reasons for doubting this suggestion.

First, although *groups* of dyslexics tend to perform worse than *groups* of normals on short-term memory tasks, once again not all dyslexics do badly. It is possible to be a dyslexic with a normal memory span, as has been shown by Torgeson and Houck (1980). Second, while it seems unlikely that poor reading could cause poor short-term memory performance, an alternative and more likely possibility is that some third factor causes association between difficulties in learning to read and problems with short-term memory tasks. For example, both could be due to a general tendency for left hemisphere functions (of which verbal short-term memory is one) to be carried out less effectively by dyslexics than normals. If it really is possible to exclude all environmental factors (like education and opportunity) as causes of dyslexia, then all that remains is some origin within the constitution of the individual. Since most language processes are the responsibility of the left hemisphere, and since the acquired dyslexias are known to arise from left hemisphere injuries, it is natural to look within that hemisphere for the presumed constitutional causes of developmental dyslexia. There is much indirect and some more direct evidence for worse average performance by dyslexics on a variety of left hemisphere mediated behaviors.

DEVELOPMENTAL DYSLEXIA AND
THE LEFT CEREBRAL HEMISPHERE

In a booklet introducing the work done on developmental dyslexia at the University of Aston in Birmingham, England, Newton and Wilsher (1979) cite the following as "diagnostic indicators" which often co-occur with developmental dyslexia:

1. Late language development (also reported by Ingram, 1963).
2. A tendency to speech errors, for example, saying "my eggs do lache" instead of "my legs do ache," and greater than average difficulty repeating long spoken words like "preliminary" or "statistical" (also noted by Miles and N. Ellis, 1981).
3. Perhaps some early signs of clumsiness and poor coordination.

To a neuropsychologist these signs are highly suggestive of left hemisphere deficits because speech and action planning are both left hemisphere skills. Object naming and verbal short-term memory also involve the left hemisphere, and are tasks on which differences between groups of dyslexics and groups of normals have been reported (see Warrington, 1967; Denckla, 1979; and Jorm, 1979). In addition, published reports suggest that dyslexics as a group are as good as normals on tasks like picture completion or object assembly which are within the scope of the right hemisphere (Miles and N. Ellis, 1981; Thomson, 1982).

Some studies have reported more direct signs of left hemisphere differences between dyslexic and normal children, for example, in the patterns of electrical activity which can be detected on the surface of the head or in the relative sizes of certain regions of cortex in the two hemispheres of the brain (see Jorm, 1979; Masland, 1981; Hughes, 1982; and Pirozzolo and Hansch, 1982 for reviews). As this book is about the cognitive psychology of reading, writing, and dyslexia we shall not go in any depth into this work other than to note that if the left hemispheres of developmental dyslexics are different from or less efficient than those of nondyslexics, then the differences that might be observed between groups of normals and dyslexics will extend beyond reading to a range of other left hemisphere skills. Evidence of an association between reading retardation and these other skills does not prove a causal link between the reading difficulty and the problems with object naming, verbal short-term memory, action sequencing, or whatever. Indeed, to discover, as Torgeson and Houck (1980) did, a group of dyslexic children with normal memory spans and object naming speeds argues strongly against such a causal link.

From time to time one encounters the claim that dyslexia research would be on a surer footing if some "objective" means of diagnosing it could be discovered, whether it be an abnormal eye movement pattern or an abnormal brainwave pattern. There are two reasons for believing this view to be misguided. First, reading backwardness seems to be a graded thing more like obesity than measles. We cannot in any simple way divide the population into those who are dyslexic and those who are not, so it would seem unlikely that there will exist any symptom or sign which will qualitatively distinguish dyslexics from nondyslexics. Second, suppose we *did* find some unusual brainwave pattern or whatever which occurred in the first 999 dyslexic children tested. Suppose, too, that the one-thousandth case was a bright, articulate teenager who, despite application and skilled tuition, had made minimal progress in learning to read and write. What if that teenager showed entirely normal brainwave patterns? Would that make him or her any less of a dyslexic? Clearly not. If we discover a discrepantly poor reader whose disability cannot be put down to inadequate opportunity or teaching, and who shows normal electrical brain activity, normal lateralization, normal eye movements when not tackling print, normal short-term memory, normal visual perception, and so on, then we must acknowledge that none of those indicators is necessarily associated with dyslexia (or whatever one cares to call it), and that dyslexia can occur without abnormalities or deficiencies in any of these characteristics and abilities. In short, whatever one goes on to do with the dyslexic children one selects, the initial criteria can only be psychological and educational, and can only relate to the failure to acquire an expected standard of literacy.

To argue as we have done that many developmental dyslexics have problems with several left hemisphere mediated skills is *not* to say that developmental dyslexics are "brain injured." We have proposed that the brain and the mind are composed of many independent but intercommunicating "modules." These modules would seem to provide the important dimensions of individual cognitive differences. Some "normal" people are spectacularly poor at drawing, at remembering melodies, at remembering the spatial layout of the environment, or at arithmetic skills. These are all abilities which can also be selectively impaired by brain injury, implying that they are the responsibility of separate brain modules, or clusters of modules. Assuming that these normal individual differences are not environmental in origin, then it would seem that nature endows us with cognitive modules operating at a range of efficiencies. It so happens that in modern Western society it doesn't really matter much if one cannot draw, or gets lost easily, and one can even get by reasonably well in many walks of life with only minimal mathematical abilities. It does matter a lot, however, if one of your inefficient modules is one of those required for learning to *read*. Illiteracy is both a stigma and an enormous inconvenience in the modern world, so developmental dyslexia causes great concern and generates large quantities of research, whereas developmental inability to draw or calculate can pass virtually unnoticed.

COMPARING DEVELOPMENTAL AND ACQUIRED DYSLEXIA

If we are on the right path in regarding developmental dyslexia as due to some relative inefficiency of left hemisphere modules, and if the acquired dyslexias are caused by injury to those same modules, then one might expect some similarities between developmental and acquired dyslexia. This is not a new idea—James Hinshelwood, whose pioneering work was mentioned earlier, drew parallels between the difficulties of dyslexic children and those of brain-injured adults. Some recent unitary approaches to this issue have sought to liken *all* or most developmental dyslexics to just one variety of acquired dyslexia. We shall look at two such proposals before going on to argue that, in fact, developmental dyslexia comes in different varieties just as acquired dyslexia does, and that there are close similarities between the two sets.

Is developmental dyslexia like acquired deep dyslexia?

In a review of the cognitive and physiological bases of developmental dyslexia, Jorm (1979) drew attention to what he considered to be important similarities between developmental dyslexia and acquired deep dyslexia. One of Jorm's points of similarity had to do with the problems that both developmental and deep dyslexics have when it comes to reading nonwords like *blint* aloud. We know from the work of Snowling (1980, 1981), Seymour and Porpodas (1980) and others that when it comes to reading nonwords, developmental dyslexics are slower and less accurate even than younger, normal children with the same reading age as the dyslexics. (Reading age is based on the number of real words a child can read aloud correctly.) However, as Baddeley, N. C. Ellis, Miles, and Lewis (1981) point out, although developmental dyslexics are undoubtedly inefficient at reading nonwords, they are not totally incapable in the way acquired deep dyslexics are.

As was reported in Chapter 4, deep dyslexics are better at reading imageable words aloud than abstract words. Jorm (1977) showed that the same was true of developmental dyslexics and listed this in his 1979 paper as another similarity between developmental and deep dyslexia. However, Baddeley, N. C. Ellis, Miles, and Lewis (1981) showed that this superiority for imageable words extended to normal children. These authors go on to suggest that abstract words may tend to be learned later than imageable words, and that age-of-acquisition may lie at the root of the so-called "imageability effect" in both normal children and developmental dyslexics.

There are other problems which arise when any strong claims to similarity between deep and developmental dyslexics are made (Ellis, 1979c), but the major stumbling block concerns the question of whether out-and-out semantic errors ever occur in developmental dyslexics. In an early paper on "linguistic lapses" Wells (1906, pp. 77–78) reports an intriguing case of a child who was taught to read entirely by the look-and-say method and who apparently made semantic errors such as misreading *corn* as "wheat," *locomotive* as "engine," and *dog* as "cat." Once again, however, we cannot be sure that Wells's child made these errors when reading words presented in isolation. We know that both skilled readers and children will make "narremic errors" when reading connected text aloud, but it has never been convincingly demonstrated that they will make these errors to words shown singly. One cannot justify claims to similarity between developmental and deep dyslexia which are based on errors made by the developmental dyslexics in text reading (cf., Critchley and Critchley, 1978, pp. 28–29).

In short, there seems to be little mileage to be had in comparing typical developmental dyslexics with acquired deep dyslexics. Certainly, until very recently there were no detailed case reports of developmental dyslexics in the literature to which one could point and say, "This may be a case of developmental deep dyslexia." The situation has changed somewhat with the publication of a recent case study by Johnston (1983).

The girl (C. R.) reported by Johnston was eighteen years old when tested, though her reading age was only six years two months. She was better reading imageable than abstract nouns and was extremely poor at reading nonwords (though, as has been noted, neither of these "symptoms" is particularly informative on its own). Of greater importance are the errors C. R. made. Over the course of several sessions, C. R. was given 382 words to read aloud. She read seventy-eight correctly and was unable to offer any response to a further 219 words. Fifty of C. R.'s errors were visual by Johnston's criterion of at least half of the letters in the error also being present in the stimulus word (examples[1] include *cigar* read as "sugar," *cost* as "cot," and *rice* as "ripe). In addition, C. R. made three possible derivational errors (e.g., *eye* read as "eyes," and *child* as "children") and nine function word substitutions (e.g., *she* read as "her," *their* as "that," and *who* as "how").

Visual errors, derivational errors, and function word substitutions all occur in deep dyslexia but are not unique to that syndrome. Most crucial of all are the five semantic errors which C. R. made to words shown singly. These were *office* read as "occupation," *down* as "up," *seven* as "eight," *chair* as "table," and *table* as "chair." Now, if you have never seen a particular word before and hazard a pure guess at what it is, then the probability of your guess bearing an entirely fortuitous semantic relationship to the target word can be surprisingly high, even in the absence of helpful context (Ellis and Marshall, 1978). This is a fact that researchers must bear in mind when testing for the occurrence of semantic errors. However, for C. R.'s semantic errors to be attributable to chance one would expect quite a number of errors which are neither visually nor semantically similar to their targets. In fact only fifteen of C. R.'s errors were neither visually nor semantically related to the target word. In addition she also made one visual-then-semantic error (*sleep* read as "lamb," presumably via "sheep"); hitherto such errors have only ever been observed in acquired deep dyslexics.

---

[1]R. Johnston, personal communication.

C. R. may be a genuine developmental deep dyslexic, but one would ideally like to see a case showing a higher incidence of semantic errors to single words. Also, C. R. suffered from a head injury when young, and one cannot be as confident as one would like to be that no brain injury occurred. This case is suggestive and will hopefully spur others on to look for less equivocal cases to establish whether or not developmental deep dyslexia genuinely exists.

Is developmental dyslexia like acquired surface dyslexia?

Where Jorm (1979) drew parallels between developmental dyslexia and acquired deep dyslexia, Holmes (1973; 1978) made the contrary claim that close similarities exist between developmental dyslexia and acquired *surface* dyslexia. Recall that surface dyslexics read predominantly phonically, and frequently arrive at a meaning for a word on the basis of its sound rather than its appearance. Often the phonemic form of the word from which its sound is generated is achieved by breaking the written form up into single letters or letter groups to which analogies or correspondencies are then applied. This strategy results in typically phonic errors; for example, regularizing *bread* to "breed" and *island* to "izland," or failing to lengthen the vowel in a word which ends in *e*, thereby reading *bike* as "bik" and *describe* as "describ" (see Chapter 4, and especially Table 4.1).

Precisely the same sorts of oral reading errors were made by the four developmental dyslexic boys, aged between nine and thirteen years, who were studied by Holmes (1973; 1978), and by a "developmental surface dyslexic" girl, C. D., reported by Coltheart (1981; 1982) and Coltheart, Masterson, Byng, Prior, and Riddoch (1983). C. D. was of normal intelligence (Verbal IQ 105, Performance IQ 101), had entirely normal speech production and comprehension, no marked defect in short-term memory as assessed by digit span, and no history or evidence of any form of neurological abnormality. Nevertheless, at the age of fifteen, despite adequate educational opportunity, her reading age was only between ten and eleven years, and her errors were quintessentially surface dyslexic. When C. D. was asked to define a word before saying it, her definition always matched her subsequent pronunciation. At the same time she could prove her problems are not of a peripheral, perceptual nature by going on to name each of the letters in the word she had just misread. For example, shown *check* C. D. responded, "part of your face . . . cheek . . . C, H, E, C, K."

The define-then-pronounce task revealed another aspect of C. D.'s dyslexia which a simple reading aloud task would almost certainly have failed to pick up. Shown *pane* C. D. said, "something which hurts . . . pain . . . P, A, N, E," and shown *bowled* she said, "fierce, big . . . bold

. . . B, O, W, L, E, D.'' The acquired surface dyslexic patient reported by Newcombe and Marshall (1982) made precisely the same sorts of "homophone confusion" error. In some cases the homophone which C. D. misinterpreted was itself an irregular word (e.g., defining *bury* as "a fruit on a tree"). This shows that C. D. sometimes obtained the phonemic form of a word on a whole-word basis—another instance of the occasional use by surface dyslexics of direct connections between visual word recognition units and phonemic word production units (cf., Chapter 4). Finally, like all surface dyslexics, C. D. was notably more successful at reading regular words aloud than irregular words.

It is an unfortunate fact that many of the difficulties experienced by C. D. and other surface dyslexics are a direct consequence of the complexities and irregularities of English spelling. A language with a more consistent alphabetic spelling system should create substantially fewer problems for acquired or developmental surface dyslexics. This point was dramatically illustrated by Coltheart (1982) in his report of a bilingual man (F. E.) who was surface dyslexic when reading English words aloud but had no difficulty reading Spanish words aloud (F. E. was of Columbian extraction). The regularity of Spanish spelling meant that F. E. was considerably more successful in his attempts to read Spanish, though he was still prone to misinterpret Spanish homophones.

C. D. is a girl of normal intelligence with a reading age four years or so below what would normally be expected of her. There is no doubt, then, that she qualifies for the label "dyslexic" (or any of the other similar terms) by the criteria outlined at the beginning of this chapter. However, we have already seen in the previous chapter that *normal* Stage Three and Four readers can resemble acquired surface dyslexics in the advantage they show for regular over irregular words, and in the sorts of errors they make. In fact, C. D.'s performance is indistinguishable from that of the normal nine- to ten-years-olds studied by Simpson (1983) and the Reading Age Controls included in Coltheart, Masterson, Byng, Prior, and Riddoch's (1983) study. It is hard to say as yet precisely what this implies, but it is at least possible that in developmental surface dyslexia we are seeing a *retardation* in the normal process of learning to read. The concept of dyslexia as a slower progression through the normal stages is one that has been proposed from time to time (e.g., Bender, 1957; Ingram, 1963; Zurif and Carson, 1970) and discussed by Holmes (1978). It *might* have some validity as applied to developmental surface dyslexia, in which case we may not need to posit specific impairments in these cases, but firm conclusions must await further research and further conceptual clarification.

Developmental phonological dyslexia

Temple and Marshall (1983) have recently produced the first detailed description of a developmental phonological dyslexic. As discussed in Chapter 4, acquired phonological dyslexics rely to a very large extent on direct visual word recognition. They read irregular words as well as they read regular words, but they are very poor at pronouncing unfamiliar words or nonwords. The real word reading of acquired phonological dyslexics is not, however, perfect as they are prone to both visual and derivational errors. They do not make semantic errors when reading single words aloud.

The seventeen-year-old developmental dyslexic girl H. M. reported by Temple and Marshall showed exactly the same pattern of abilities and disabilities. H. M.'s IQ, memory span, and command of the spoken language were quite normal but her reading age was only around ten or eleven. She was as good at reading irregular words as regular words though she made both visual errors (e.g., *cheery* read as "cherry," *bouquet* as "boutique," and *attractive* as "achieve"), and derivational errors (e.g., *cautious* read as "caution," *appeared* as "appearance," and *smoulder* as "smouldering").

H. M.'s reading of nonwords and real, but uncommon words was very poor. When presented with ten very simple three-letter nonwords she still manged to read four incorrectly (*gok* read as "joke," *bix* as "back," *nup* as "nap," and *hib* as "hip"). These errors illustrate H. M.'s tendency to use the strategy of approximate visual access and to read nonwords as real words. In fact about two-thirds of her errors to nonwords were of this type. Even her nonwords responses look rather wordlike, for example *cenectricities* read as "cenelectricals," and *lumilination* as "limitinations."

We have suggested that C. D., the developmental surface dyslexic discussed in the previous section, may have become stuck at the level of reading ability typical of a normal nine- or ten-year-old. We have also noted in Chapter 7 the similarity between young children in Stages 1 and 2 of Marsh *et al.'s* developmental sequence and acquired phonological dyslexics. Is it possible that, in terms of functional reading skills, H. M. has remained fixated at such an early stage in the normal process of learning to read? Was she a normal reader up to the age of six or seven when her peers began to develop phonic skills and she did not? An alternative approach is to argue that, just as the visual word recognition system and grapheme-phoneme conversion can be differentially impaired by brain injury, so one can be differentially endowed by nature with the capacity to develop these two modules. Once again, this cognitive-neuropsychological approach is such a recent development that, while one may feel that we are now beginning to ask the right questions, we can unfortunately provide few of the answers.

Developmental letter-by-letter (spelling) dyslexia?

In Hinshelwood's (1917) *Congenital Word-Blindness* can be found a number of case studies of dyslexic children. Here is one such case study:

> a boy, 12 years of age, was brought in March 1902 to the Glasgow Eye Infirmary by his mother, to see if there was anything wrong with his eyesight. . . . On examining him I found that his reading was very defective for a boy who had been seven years at school. He could rarely read by sight more than two or three words, and was unable to proceed unless he was allowed to spell the word aloud . . . or to spell it silently with his lips. The words he stuck at were chiefly polysyllables, but this was not always the case, as he often failed to recognize by sight even simple monosyllabic words. He spelt very well, and when asked to spell the words which he had failed to recognize by sight, he nearly always did so without any difficulty. . . . He was strong in arithmetic, good at spelling, and average in other subjects, including geography and history. (Hinshelwood, 1917, pp. 49–51)

Extracting the principal points, we see that this boy seems to have been reasonably intelligent, being good at arithmetic and average at other subjects. His reading was slow and tortuous and he frequently resorted to saying the letter names aloud or to himself before identifying a word. His written spelling, in contrast, was good. The similarity between this boy's pattern of abilities and inabilities and what the turn of the century neurologists used to call "alexia without agraphia" was not lost on Hinshelwood. We have met alexia without agraphia in Chapter 5, although there we called it by the more recent name "letter-by-letter reading," (alias "word-form dyslexia" or "spelling dyslexia"). This plethora of terms is confusing but unimportant—what matters is that we have here a developmental dyslexic boy whose symptoms are quite unlike those shown by any of the dyslexic children described earlier in this chapter, but closely resemble a well-known variety of acquired dyslexia.

In Chapter 5 we argued that acquired letter-by-letter dyslexics had either lost access to the visual word recognition system or had lost that system itself and were, as a consequence, obliged to read by using a graphemic code to trigger graphemic word production units in the spelling system. The boy described by Hinshelwood was a developmental dyslexic whose problems, if our theory is correct, was that he had great difficulty in *forming* visual word recognition units. (It appears from the account given that he could recognize a few words "by sight", that is, through the triggering of hard-won recognition units.) However, his competence in spelling implies a normal capacity to develop graphemic word production units which permitted him to read after a fashion through the tortuous device of pronouncing individual letter names.

Hyperlexia

Developmental dyslexia refers to a condition in which otherwise intelligent children unexpectedly fail to learn to read. It would appear that sometimes the opposite pattern occurs; that is, backward, retarded children develop a surprising and unexpected *ability* to read aloud. This phenomenon has been term "hyperlexia."

One of the cases described by Silberberg and Silberberg (1968) concerns a second-grade (nine-year-old) boy with a measured IQ of only sixty-four (far below normal) whose expressive speech was poorly developed, but who nevertheless was able to read words to a third-grade (ten-year-old) level. Significantly, Silberberg and Silberberg (1968, p. 5) add that, "Of course, his comprehension of what he read was commensurate with his measured intelligence."

The first of three children described by Huttenlocher and Huttenlocher (1973) is a seven-year-old boy (M. K.) with an IQ of only seventy-seven and with speech and motor development equivalent to that of a normal three and a half-year-old child. At the age of two "he learned nursery rhymes and television commercials with remarkable facility, but he had great difficulty in learning to associate names with objects in picture books" (p. 1108). Between four and four and a half years he learned to read "with minimal parental help" and at the age of four years ten months he is described as having read fluently a passage appropriate for a normal ten-year-old.

In M. K. and comparable hyperlexic children the skill of reading aloud has developed to a level beyond the child's other cognitive abilities. There are hints, too, that reading aloud outstrips comprehension and that the hyperlexic child may fail to understand material that he or she nevertheless reads aloud successfully. Does this pattern in hyperlexia have a counterpart in any of the acquired dyslexias? While it would be unwise to press the comparison too hard at this stage, there are obvious similarities between the symptoms of the particular hyperlexic children just discussed (who, to repeat, are not representative of all children dubbed "hyperlexic") and the syndrome of acquired "direct dyslexia" discussed in Chapter 4.

It will be recalled that the direct dyslexic patient W. L. P. suffered a progressive presenile dementia which gradually robbed her of virtually all *understanding* of spoken or written language. She was still capable, however, of reading aloud many words, a skill which was ascribed in Chapter 4 to the intactness of direct connections between visual word recognition units and phonemic word production units (hence the phrase "direct dyslexia"). Is it possible that hyperlexic children also read aloud by means of such intact connections without any necessary intervention of comprehension and semantic codes? Such a suggestion is close in spirit to the account of hyperlexia given by Huttenlocher and Huttenlocher (1973).

Huttenlocher and Huttenlocher propose that familiar words are recognized by "visual schema" (the equivalent of our visual word recognition units). Visual schema connect to word concepts (our semantic representations), and also, separately, to "auditory schema" (our phonemic word production units). Huttenlocher and Huttenlocher (p. 1114) note that in hyperlexics like M. K., "The observed deficit would . . . seem to be . . . a diminished ability to associate word schemas with their meanings" (see also Richman and Kitchell, 1981, and Healy, 1982). Despite this deficit, reading aloud is still possible by virtue of the direct connections between visual schemas and auditory schemas.

Hyperlexic children are also typically good at reading nonwords phonically; thus Huttenlocher and Huttenlocher (p. 1108) tell us that M. K.'s mother "first discovered that he could sound out words when he read "SNOINO" on a can which had "ONIONS" printed on it and which was standing upside down." It is unlikely that hyperlexic reading is *predominantly* phonic since there is no mention of any specific problems with irregular words in hyperlexics. This fact does not, however, invalidate the comparison with acquired direct dyslexia because although we are not provided with any details of phonic reading in W. L. P., Schwartz, Saffran, and Marin (1980) claim that she could successfully pronounce written nonwords. There may be supporting evidence here for the idea mooted in Chapter 4 that direct connections between visual word recognition units and phonemic word production units play a role in analogy-based phonic reading.

THE VARIETIES OF DEVELOPMENTAL DYSLEXIA

If we put hyperlexia on one side, then we have still identified putative cases of four different varieties of developmental dyslexia, specifically:

1. Developmental deep dyslexia
2. Developmental surface dyslexia
3. Developmental phonological dyslexia
4. Developmental letter-by-letter reading.

The status of developmental deep dyslexia is still doubtful, and Hinshelwood's report of developmental letter-by-letter reading is the only one the author is aware of, suggesting that it is probably a very rare syndrome (and again we cannot yet exclude the possibility of early brain injury). Those few studies of groups of developmental dyslexics which have looked for individual differences in the actual reading strategies used suggest that most developmental dyslexics are of the surface type (like C. D.) or the phonological type (like H. M.), or show a combination of both types of symptoms.

Mitterer's (1982) division of poor readers into whole-word and recoding types

Mitterer (1982) examined the reading strategies of twenty-seven eight-year-old "poor readers" and isolated ten who relied predominantly on whole-word recognition of words by sight ("whole-word" readers equivalent to developmental phonological dyslexia) and a further ten who relied predominantly on phonic mediation ("recoding" readers equivalent to developmental surface dyslexia). These two groups differed in their performance on a number of tasks though they were indistinguishable on overall IQ or even IQ subtest scores, and indistinguishable too on a standardized reading test.

The recoders read substantially more regular than irregular words correctly, as one would expect of readers capable of using the phonic route. Whole-word dyslexics, in contrast, showed no such difference. If a word was within their sight vocabulary they could read it, whether regular or irregular. If it was outside their sight vocabulary they could not read it, so could not boost their scores by successfully sounding out an additional few regular words. The errors of recoders to real words were predominantly phonic ("Conservative" in Mitterer's terminology) and included a substantial proportion of nonwords. The errors of whole-word dyslexics, on the other hand, were predominantly visual ("Liberal" in Mitterer's terminology) and included very few nonwords. Similarly, recoders gave regular pronunciations to nonwords and read few of them as real words whereas whole-word readers tended not to give the expected regular pronunciations to nonwords and instead read many as real words.

Boder's (1971; 1973) distinction between dyseidetic and dysphonetic dyslexics

A distinction similar to that between whole-word readers and decoders was made by Boder (1971; 1973). The whole-word (phonological) type Boder called *dysphonetic dyslexics*. These children were said to possess a limited sight vocabulary of words which they were able to recognize visually, but to be very poor at phonic decoding. The errors made by dysphonetic dyslexics were often visual, for example, reading *house* as "horse," *money* as "monkey," or *step* as "stop." Boder also claims that dysphonetic dyslexics make semantic errors such as reading *laugh* as "funny," *duck* as "chicken," or *moon* as "planet," but these may have narremic substitutions made to words in sentences rather than semantic errors made to words in isolation.

The decoding (surface) type of poor reader Boder called *dyseidetic dyslexics*. According to Boder (1973, p. 670) the dyseidetic dyslexic "reads laboriously, as if he is seeing each word for the first time. . . . He is an *analytic* reader and reads 'by ear', through a process of phonetic analysis and synthesis, sounding out familiar as well as unfamiliar combinations of letters." Typical errors of the dyseidetic dyslexic include *laugh* read as "log" or "loge," *business* as "bussyness," and *talk* as "talc."

The EXPECTED nature of individual differences among poor (and good) readers

Having just surveyed some recent attempts to distinguish varieties of developmental dyslexia, we shall now draw upon the treatment of reading and acquired dyslexia in the earlier chapters in order to ask what form we should *expect* individual differences among both poor and normal readers to take. Let us begin by reiterating a point made in Chapter 4 when we were considering varieties of acquired dyslexia. The point made there was that the individual patients reported as cases of surface dyslexia, deep dyslexia, or whatever tend to be the exceptional patients who have a particularly "pure" form of reading disorder. Most patients will have a mixture of reading problems, combined with problems processing spoken language, but the claim (or at least the hope) is that the problems of the average patient will be explicable as a particular combination of the pure forms of dyslexia and aphasia.

Anyone coming to the study of developmental dyslexia from a background in cognitive psychology and neuropsychology would anticipate a similar situation. If we restrict ourselves to those individual differences captured by the distinction between phonic and whole-word skills, what would we expect? We might expect to find an occasional individual with normal direct, visual word recognition but very poor phonic skills. Such an individual would *not*, however, qualify as dyslexic because reading age is normally assessed from real-word reading. The sort of person we have in mind would probably be diagnosed in Baron and Strawson's (1976) terms as a "Chinese" reader—someone who relies heavily on whole-word visual identification.

In addition to the Chinese readers, Baron and Strawson (1976) identify a subgroup of normal "Phoenecian" readers. These people (students in the study in question) rely more heavily than the average reader on phonic mediation. Their visual whole-word identification cannot be too substandard or they would presumably never have achieved college status, but they still are towards the surface dyslexic-type end of the normal spectrum. What is important to appreciate is that extreme Chinese and Phoenecian readers are rare animals. The normal pattern is for a person to be good, mediocre, or poor at both whole-word and phonic processing.

Turning to the clear developmental dyslexics, Temple and Marshall (1983) have shown that their developmental phonological dyslexic girl H. M. was far worse at phonic than whole-word processes, but even her whole-word processes must have been below what one would expect from her age and IQ or she would have been a normal Chinese reader rather than a developmental dyslexic. Similarly, Coltheart, Masterson, Byng, Prior, and Riddoch (1983) show that the developmental surface dyslexic girl C. D. showed poor visual whole-word identification but some capacity for phonic mediation, but the evidence discussed earlier implies that C. D.'s phonic skills are only what one would expect from her reading age, not what one would expect from her actual chronological age. (She was *not* a normal Phoenecian reader.)

So, in H. M. and C. D. we are looking at *relative* not absolute development of differential whole-word and phonic word recognition skills. H. M.'s whole-word identification was better than her phonic skills but was still not normal, and C. D.'s phonic abilities may have determined her predominant reading strategy but they too may only have been relatively well developed.

When Boder (1973) tested 107 dyslexic children she estimated that sixty-seven fell into the dysphonetic (alias phonological or whole-word) type and ten into the dyseidetic (alias surface or recoding) type. Two points are worth making here. The first is that only a few of Boder's dysphonetic dyslexics are likely to have been as pure as Temple and Marshall's H. M. and only a few of her dyseidetic dyslexics as pure as Coltheart *et al's* C. D. Boder's classification (like Mitterer's) is in terms of relative development and reliance on whole-word or phonic routes. (In fact, Boder classifies her dyslexics on the spelling rather than reading.) The second point is that twenty-seven of Boder's dyslexics were classed as mixed "dysphonetic-dyseidetic dyslexics"—children who had roughly equal (and severe) problems with both routes. Similarly, seven of Mitterer's poor readers seem to have shown equal difficulties with whole-word and recoding processes. According to Boder these are the children who had the greatest difficulty ever achieving any degree of functional literacy.

All the work cited here has sought to distinguish among readers on the basis of components and strategies of normal reading. There have been other attempts at distinguishing reading subgroups, for example, on the basis of their scores on standardized neuropsychological or intelligence test batteries (see Vernon, 1979; Satz and Morris, 1981; and Malatesha and Aaron, 1982, for reviews and examples), but the approach advocated here is that which has proved so successful in distinguishing varieties of normal and acquired dyslexic readers; that is, typology based on observed patterns of relatively intact and impaired reading processes and components. Note that we must expect most dyslexics, whether developmental or acquired, to have mixed disabilities though they may be more biased toward one type than another. We should not be surprised either when groups of developmental dyslexics show impairment of many different aspects of reading when compared with normals. Pure forms of a particular syndrome should occur from time to time, but they will be the exception rather than the rule. The fact that dyslexics do not all fall neatly into one or other of the proposed subtypes is not an argument against the validity of those types.

We may note in passing that both direct visual word recognition and phonically mediated recognition are left hemisphere skills for almost all right-handed people, and for most left-handers too. The right hemisphere of the brain may develop a limited capacity for whole-word identification, but that system is at best subordinate to that of the left hemisphere (Coltheart, 1983). There is no basis whatsoever for arguing as some have done that dysphonetic (whole-word) dyslexics may have left hemisphere deficits while dyseidetic (recoding) dyslexics must have right hemisphere deficits. If these developmental problems in acquiring literacy are indeed rooted in the brains of those afflicted, then their language-dominant hemispheres, which will usually be their left hemispheres, must be the culprits in both cases.

DYSLEXIC SPELLING AND WRITING

Such research as has been done on the cognitive psychology of developmental dyslexia has very much tended to focus on reading rather spelling. This is perhaps a little surprising when one considers that it is the poor writing of dyslexics which is often noticed first, and that spelling problems often persist in "ex-dyslexics" who have achieved a passable degree of reading skill (Critchley and Critchley, 1978).

Miles (1983) provides an interesting corpus and classification of dyslexic spelling errors. Some of the errors are phonic (e.g., *GOWING* for *going*, *ECODE* for *echoed*) or "misfired" phonic attempts (e.g., *WHIV* for *with*, *YUWER* for *your*), but a great many, when pronounced, would not sound like the target word. Some spelling errors have all of the letters but in the wrong order (e.g., *PAKR* for *park*, *THRID* for *third*, *ESLE* for *else*, and *SONW* for *snow*). Miles proposes that the much-quoted "kinetic reversal" spelling errors like *WAS* for *saw* or *ON* for *no* should be subsumed within this larger category of errors. Knowing the letters but not the order would seem to qualify as having partial information about a word's spelling—a phenomenon we discussed in Chapter 5. Two adult developmental dyslexics reported by Seymour and Porpodas (1980) made this sort of error, particularly when trying to spell fairly common words which they knew to be irregular, for example spelling *sword* as *SOWRD*, *tongue* as *TOUNGE*, or *muscle* as *MUCLE*. This last error lacks one of the letters of a target but must count as an example of the retrieval of partial information from the speller's graphemic word production system, as must a number of the other errors listed by Miles (1983), for example, *mechanical* misspelled as *MECHINAL* (note the *CH* for /k/), *write* as *WRTE* (the *W*), *people* as *PEPEOLE* (the *O*), and *language* as *LANGUAGUGE* (just about everything!).

Miles's corpus is collected from many dyslexics over many years, but does not tell us whether individual dyslexic children vary in the extent to which they are disposed to produce different sorts of error. Boder (1973) proposes that they do indeed, and that dyseidetic, dysphonetic, and mixed dyslexics can be distinguished on their spelling patterns as well as on their reading patterns. Dyseidetic (alias developmental surface) dyslexics, whose reading relies heavily on phonic mediation, are said to also spell phonically. Examples provided by Boder include *LAF* for *laugh*, *BURD* for *bird*, *HOWS* for *house*, and *VAKASHN* for *vacation*. C. D., the sixteen-year-old developmental surface dyslexic girl discussed earlier, also spelled phonically, for instance, misspelling "search" as *SURCH* and "capacity" as *CAPASATY*, though in addition she made some errors which were not phonic and which showed evidence of partial spelling knowledge, for instance misspelling "cough" as *COULG* and "exaggerate" as *EXADERT*. Once again, we might note that these surface dyslexic spelling errors would be quite normal in younger children of the same spelling age and are only "dyslexic" by virtue of the age, intelligence, and education of the perpetrator.

Developmental dysphonetic (alias phonological) dyslexics are sight readers whose phonic reading is very poor. If their spelling were similar then we would expect them to have a certain capacity for spelling from memory but to be very poor at assembling spellings from sounds. This seems to have been the case for Boder's dysphonetic dyslexics. According to Boder the typical dysphonetic dyslexic "cannot spell phonetically. He spells correctly to dictation only those words in his sight vocabulary. . . .

Typically the correctly written words are islands in a sea of dysphonetic mis-spelling" (Boder, 1973, p. 669). Errors produced by dysphonetic dyslexics include *CATTEGT* for *cottage*, *COETERE* for *character*, and *SLEBER* for *scrambled*. As Boder acknowledges, these are not entirely random misspellings (e.g., the first letter is correct in each case), but they are far less accurate phonically than the errors of the dyseidetic dyslexics.

Boder (1973) seems to assume that the reading and spelling patterns of a dyslexic will always complement one another. We have already seen that this is not necessarily true for patients with acquired reading and spelling disorders. For example, the patient R. G. discussed in Chapter 5 was a phonological dyslexic but a surface dysgraphic; that is, he read predominantly "by eye," but spelled predominantly "by ear." We have met this pattern before in Bryant and Bradley's (1980) six-year-olds, and it also occurs in older people who are good readers but very poor spellers (most people will be able to number at least one such individual among their acquaintances). Frith (1978; 1980a) has shown that people who are good readers but poor spellers are actually "Chinese" sight readers but "Phoenecian" phonic spellers. They are not developmental dyslexics, but one might make out a case for calling them developmental dysgraphics.

H. M., Temple and Marshall's (1983) developmental phonological dyslexic, was very poor at phonic reading but good at phonic spelling. When tested at the age of seventeen she spelled at the normal ten-year-old level, but over half her errors were phonic (e.g. *SOLOM* for *solemn*, *CHEET* for *cheat*, and *MATRESS* for *mattress*). She was also more successful at spelling regular than irregular words, which means that she was unlike Boder's dysphonetic dyslexics and like the patient R. G. in her combination of phonological dyslexia and surface dysgraphia. Where H. M.'s errors deviated from being phonic it was often because they incorporated some partial knowledge of the word's spelling (e.g., *AURDENCE* for *audience*, and *CHORCE* for *chorus*. Just as most of H. M.'s correct spellings must have originated from her graphemic word production system, so some of her errors contained letters originating from imperfectly registered items in that same store.

One important lesson of H. M. is that the reading and spelling strategies of a dyslexic individual must be assessed and diagnosed separately. Because a child or adult is a dysphonetic reader it does not automatically follow that he or she will be a dysphonetic speller. (As yet we have no data on the frequency with which different patterns of reading and spelling disability co-occur.) Also, one should not go away with the impression that one or other of whole-word or phonic spelling is always relatively intact in dyslexic spellers. Boder's (1973) group of mixed dysphonetic-dyslexic dyslexics were extremely bad at both whole-word and phonic spelling (resembling acquired "amnestic" dysgraphics in this regard). The misspellings of these children may bear little or no resemblence to the target word (e.g., writing *JE* for *to*, or *LEK* for *little*).

Finally, developmental dyslexics usually write poorly in the sense of showing poor execution of even those words which can be spelled correctly. Descriptions and samples of dyslexic handwriting can be found in Orton (1931), Hermann and Voldby (1946), and Critchley and Critchley (1978). Hermann and Voldby note among other things the similarity between certain characteristic dyslexic errors, such as the tendency to fuse adjacent letters into one, and some of the types of slip of the pen observed in normal adults. This may be one of those many cases where a dysfunction shows itself as a heightened tendency to errors which normal people are also prone to make involuntarily.

TEACHING DYSLEXICS

Finally we come to the question of teaching developmental dyslexics. The first point to be made is that dyslexic children will, in the main, respond to help. Hornsby and Miles (1980) showed that dyslexic children's rate of learning to read and spell improved dramatically once they began to receive specialist help. The children received their help in centres which varied to some degrees in the programs they used, but had in common the fact that they "all took the concept of dyslexia seriously."

Naidoo (1981) summarizes and reviews some of the most widely used teaching schemes for dyslexic children. Though they differ in their particulars, they have several features in common. First, they teach reading, writing, and relevant language skills; there is no evidence to show that having children crawl around on the floor (or restricting the use of one side of the body, or discouraging "right hemisphere" activities such as the enjoyment of music) has any effect on their reading and writing. Second, all the widely used methods are highly structured, taking children slowly and cumulatively through a detailed series of tasks and exercises. Third, in Naidoo's (1981) words, "All employ a phonic approach and all eschew whole-word methods."

Why this bias towards phonics? Because, if Boder's (1973) figures are generalizable, then the majority of dyslexic children lean towards the dysphonetic type, having at least some capacity for visual whole-word recognition but very limited phonic skills. On the assumption that one should teach to a pupil's weaknesses rather than his or her strengths, then dysphonetic dyslexics should benefit from structured phonic teaching. Even dyseidetic dyslexics may in fact be relying on somewhat deficient skills of phonic recoding which could be improved by further training.

Another point which we have already made earlier is that whereas whole-word or look-and-say methods tutor only the direct, visual reading route, phonic methods probably tutor both routes since recognition units will be established eventually for the words used to illustrate the various phonic correspondences and procedures.

At the same time one would predict that the characteristics of the individual dyslexic child will to some extent determine which teaching methods will prove most effective. An extreme dysphonetic dyslexic may be incapable of ever developing more than the most rudimentary phonic skills. In this case one might be better advised to teach to the dyslexic's strengths by using whole-word and sentence based methods. Paradoxically, an extreme dyseidetic dyslexic may learn phonic recoding rapidly but may also benefit from word-specific help in learning to identify visually those irregular and inconsistent words which resist rational decoding. Boder (1973) claims that dysphonetic dyslexics benefit most from initial whole-word techniques (presumably to develop Stage One and Two capabilities), with phonics only being introduced when the child has acquired a sufficient sight vocabulary. Phonic methods are advocated from the start for dyseidetic children, presumably on the grounds that sight recognition will develop as a natural side-effect of this approach. It should be noted, however, that these recommendations are based purely on Boder's own experience. As yet we lack any large-scale studies looking at the extent to which individual differences between dyslexics (or normal children for that matter) may affect how they respond to different teaching methods.

SUMMARY OF CHAPTER 8

Reading ability is not entirely predictable from age and IQ. Some children of normal or above-normal intelligence have difficulty learning to read and write despite adequate backgrounds and educational opportunities. These are the children sometimes called "dyslexic," though reading ability is a graded thing and it is an arbitrary matter where one draws the line between "dyslexics" and "nondyslexics." Reading (and writing) are also dependent on several component subskills which can be separately impaired to varying degrees in developmental dyslexics, just as they can be in acquired dyslexics. Attempts to explain dyslexia as a unitary phenomenon with a single cause have therefore proved unsatisfactory. Often these explanations have been based on an observed association between reading retardation and some other difficulty where it can plausibly be argued that both are the separate results of a more general left hemisphere deficiency.

Several different varieties of developmental dyslexia have been reported, all of which resemble forms of acquired dyslexia. Developmental phonological dyslexics, otherwise known as dysphonetic or whole-word dyslexics, can learn to recognize words by sight but are very poor at phonic decoding and mediation. Developmental surface dyslexics, otherwise known as dyseidetic or recoding dyslexics, are poor at direct visual recognition and rely extensively on phonic recoding and mediation. Mixed dyseidetic-dysphonetic dyslexics have severe difficulties with both strategies of word recognition. Between them, these three varieties probably account for all but a few developmental dyslexics, though possible cases of developmental deep dyslexia and developmental letter-by-letter reading have been described. In addition some retarded children show an unexpected ability to read aloud, though they appear to comprehend little of what they read. The reading performance of at least some of these "hyperlexic" children may resemble that seen in the syndrome of "direct dyslexia" which sometimes accompanies presenile dementia.

Developmental dyslexics are also developmental dysgraphics in that their spelling is usually as bad as, if not worse than their reading. Once again, varieties or subtypes appear to exist. Developmental surface dyslexics appear to rely heavily on phonic assembly in spelling as well as in reading. Many developmental phonological dyslexics also appear to be phonological dysgraphics who are very poor at phonic spelling, but one case on record (H. M.) combines developmental phonological dyslexia with developmental surface dysgraphia; that is, she reads "by eye" but spells "by ear." The same pattern is found in good readers who are unexpectedly poor spellers.

When it comes to teaching developmental dyslexics, "phonic" methods seem to be most successful. This may be because these methods tutor both reading and spelling routes whereas whole-word methods tutor only reading by eye and spelling from memory. Boder (1973) has claimed that different types of development dyslexic respond best to different teaching methods, but this claim has yet to be formally tested.

References

Alegria, J., Pignot, E., and Morais, J. Phonetic analysis of speech and memory codes in beginning readers. *Memory and Cognition*, 1982, *10*, 451–456.

Allen, J. Speech synthesis from text. In J. C. Simon (Ed.), *Spoken Language Generation and Understanding*. Dortrecht: D. Reidel, 1980.

Allport, D. A. On knowing the meaning of words we are unable to report: the effects of visual masking. In S. Dornic (Ed.), *Attention and Performance 6*. Hillsdale, N.J.: Lawrence Erlbaum Associates, 1977.

Allport, D. A. Patterns and actions: cognitive mechanisms are content-specific. In G. Claxton (Ed.), *Cognitive psychology: New directions*. London: Routledge and Kegan Paul, 1980.

Allport, D. A. and Funnell, E. Components of the mental lexicon. *Philosophical Transactions of the Royal Society of London B*, 1981, *295*, 397–410.

Baddeley, A. D., Ellis, N. C., Miles, T. R., and Lewis, V. J. Developmental and acquired dyslexia: A comparison. *Cognition*, 1982, *11*, 185–199.

Baddeley, A. D., Eldridge, M., and Lewis, V. The role of subvocalisation in reading. *Quarterly Journal of Experimental Psychology*, 1981, *33A*, 439–454.

Baker, R. G. Orthographic awareness. In U. Frith (Ed.), *Cognitive Processes in Spelling*. London: Academic Press, 1980.

Baron, J. and Strawson, C. Use of orthographic and word-specific knowledge in reading words aloud. *Journal of Experimental Psychology: Human Perception and Performance*, 1976, *2*, 386–393.

Baron, J., Treiman, R., Wilf, J. F., and Kellman, P. Spelling and reading by rules. In U. Frith (Ed.), *Cognitive Processes in Spelling*. London: Academic Press, 1980.

Barr, R. The effect of instruction on pupil reading strategies. *Reading Research Quarterly*, 1974, *10*, 555–582.

Barron, R. W. Visual-orthographic and phonological strategies in reading and spelling. In U. Frith (Ed.), *Cognitive Processes in Spelling*. London: Academic Press, 1980.

Bastian, H. C.   On the various forms of loss of speech in cerebral disease. *British and Foreign Medico-Chirurgical Review*, 1869, *43*, 209–236 and 470–492.

Bawden, H. H.   A study of lapses. *Psychological Review Monograph Supplements*, 1900, *3*, 1–121.

Beauvois, M.-F. and Dérousné, J.   Phonological alexia: three dissociations. *Journal of Neurology, Neurosurgery and Psychiatry*, 1979, *42*, 1115–1124.

Beauvois, M.-F. and Dérousné, J.   Lexical or orthographic dysgraphia. *Brain*, 1981, *104*, 21–50.

Bender, L.   Specific reading disability as a maturational lag. *Bulletin of the Orton Society*, 1957, *7*, 9–18.

Benton, A. L. and Pearl, D. (Eds.),   *Dyslexia: An Appraisal of Current Knowledge*. New York: Oxford University Press, 1978.

Biemiller, A.   The development of the use of graphic and contextual information as children learn to read. *Reading Research Quarterly*, 1970, *6*, 75–96.

Boder, E.   Developmental dyslexia: Prevailing diagnostic concepts and a new diagnostic approach. In H. R. Myklebust (Ed.), *Progress in Learning Disabilities, Vol. 2*. New York: Grune and Stratton, 1971.

Boder, E.   Developmental dyslexia: A diagnostic approach based on three atypical reading-spelling patterns. *Developmental Medicine and Child Neurology*, 1973, *15*, 663–687.

Bradley, L.   *Assessing Reading Difficulties: A Diagnostic and Remedial Approach*. London: Macmillan Education Ltd., 1980.

Bradley, L. and Bryant, P. E.   Categorising sounds and learning to read: A causal connection. *Nature*, 1983, *301*, 419–421.

Brainerd, C. J. and Plessey, M. J. (Eds.),   *Verbal Processes in Children*. New York: Springer-Verlag, 1982.

Bransford, J. D.   *Human Cognition*. New York: Wadworth, 1979.

Bryant, P. E. and Bradley, L.   Why children sometimes write words which they do not read. In U. Frith (Ed.), *Cognitive Processes in Spelling*. London: Academic Press, 1980.

Bub, D. and Kertesz, A.   Deep agraphia. *Brain and Language*, 1982, *17*, 146–165.

Buswell, G. T.   An experimental study of eye-voice span in reading. *Supplementary Educational Monographs, No. 17*. Chicago: University of Chicago, Department of Education, 1920.

Butterworth, B.   Hesitation and semantic planning in speech. *Journal of Psycholinguistic Research*, 1975, *4*, 74–87.

Butterworth, B.   Hesitation and the production of verbal paraphasias and neologisms in jargon aphasia. *Brain and Language*, 1979, *8*, 133–161.

Campbell, R.   Writing nonwords to dictation. *Brain and Language*, 1983, *19*, 153–178.

Chall, J.   *Learning to Read: The Great Debate*. New York: McGraw-Hill, 1967.

Chomsky, C.   Reading, writing and phonology. *Harvard Educational Review*, 1970, *40*, 287–309.

Chomsky, N.   Phonology and reading. In H. Levin and J. P. Williams (Eds.), *Basic Studies on Reading*. New York: Basic Books, 1970.

Chomsky, N. and Halle, M.   *The Sound Pattern of English*. New York: Harper and Row, 1968.

Ciuffreda, K. J., Bahill, A. T., Kenyon, R. V., and Stark, L.   Eye movements during reading: Case reports. *American Journal of Optometry and Physiological Optics*, 1976, *53*, 389–395.

Collins, A. and Gentner, D.   A framework for a cognitive theory of writing. In L. W. Gregg and E. R. Steinberg (Eds.), *Cognitive Processes in Writing*. Hillsdale, N.J.: Lawrence Erlbaum, 1980.

Coltheart, M.   When can children learn to read—And when should they be taught? In T. G. Waller and G. E. Mackinnon (Eds.), *Reading Research: Advances in Theory and Practice, Vol. 1*. New York: Academic Press, 1979.

Coltheart, M.   Reading, phonological recoding, and deep dyslexia. In M. Coltheart, K. E. Patterson and J. C. Marshall (Eds.), *Deep Dyslexia*. London: Routledge and Kegan Paul, 1980 (a).

Coltheart, M.   Deep dyslexia: a right hemisphere hypothesis. In M. Coltheart, K. E. Patterson and J. C. Marshall (Eds.), *Deep Dyslexia*. London: Routledge and Kegan Paul, 1980 (b).

Coltheart, M.   Disorders of reading and their implications for models of normal reading. *Visible Language*, 1981, *15*, 245–286.

Coltheart, M.   The psycholinguistic analysis of acquired dyslexias: some illustrations. In D. E. Broadbent and L. Weiskrantz (Eds.), *The Neuropsychology of Cognitive Function*. London: The Royal Society, 1982.

Coltheart, M.   The right hemisphere and disorders of reading. In A. W. Young (Ed.), *Functions of the Right Hemisphere*. London: Academic Press, 1983.

Coltheart, M., Besner, D., Jonasson, J. T., and Davelaar, E.   Phonological encoding in the lexical decision task. *Quarterly Journal of Experimental Psychology*, 1979, *31*, 489–507.

Coltheart, M., Masterson, J., Byng, S., Prior, M., and Riddoch, J. Surface dyslexia. *Quarterly Journal of Experimental Psychology*, 1983, *35A*, 469-495.

Coltheart, M., Patterson, K. E., and Marshall, J. C. (Eds.), *Deep Dyslexia*. London: Routledge and Kegan Paul, 1980.

Critchley, M.   Specific developmental dyslexia.   In E. H. Lenneberg and E. Lenneberg (Eds.), *Foundations of Language Development, Vol. 2*. New York: Academic Press, 1975.

Critchley, M. and Critchley, E. A.   *Dyslexia Defined*. London: William Heinemann Medical Books, 1978.

Danks, J. H. and Glucksberg, S.   Experimental psycholinguistics. *Annual Review of Psychology*, 1980, *31*, 391–417.

Denckla, M. B. Childhood learning disabilities. In K. M. Heilman and E. Valenstein (Eds.), *Clinical Neuropsychology*. New York: Oxford University Press, 1979.

Dérousné, J. and Beauvois, M. F.   Phonological processing in reading: Data from alexia. *Journal of Neurology, Neurosurgery and Psychiatry*, 1979, *42*, 1125–1132.

Desberg, P., Elliott, D. E., and Marsh, G.   American Black English and spelling. In U. Frith (Ed.), *Cognitive Processes in Spelling*. London: Academic Press, 1980.

Diringer, D.   *Writing*. London: Thames and Hudson, 1962.

Doctor, E. A.   Studies on reading comprehension in children and adults. Unpublished Ph.D thesis, University of London, 1978.

Dodd, B.   The spelling abilities of profoundly pre-lingually deaf children. In U. Frith (Ed.), *Cognitive Processes in Spelling*. London: Academic Press, 1980.

Douse, T. le M.   A study of misspellings and related mistakes. *Mind*, 1900, *9*, 85–93.

Downing, J.   *Comparative Reading*. New York: Macmillan, 1973.

Downing, J. and Leong, C. K.   *Psychology of Reading*. New York: Macmillan, 1982.

Ehrlich, S. F.   Children's word recognition in prose context. *Visible Language*, 1981, *15*, 219–244.

Ellis, A. W.   Speech production and short-term memory. In J. Morton and J. C. Marshall (Eds.), *Psycholinguistics Series Vol. 2: Structures and Processes*. London: Elek Science and Cambridge, Mass: MIT Press, 1979 (a).

Ellis, A. W.   Slips of the pen. *Visible Language*, 1979, *13*, 265–282 (b).

Ellis, A. W.   Developmental and acquired dyslexia: some observations on Jorm (1979). *Cognition*, 1979, *7*, 413–420 (c)

Ellis, A. W.   Modality-specific repetition priming of auditory word recognition. *Current Psychological Research*, 1982, *2*, 123–128 (a)

Ellis, A. W. (Ed.),   *Normality and Pathology in Cognitive Functions*. London: Academic Press, 1982 (b).

Ellis, A. W. Spelling and writing (and reading and speaking). In A. W. Ellis (Ed.), *Normality and Pathology in Cognitive Functions*. London: Academic Press, 1982 (c).

Ellis, A. W. and Marshall, J. C. Semantic errors or statistical flukes? A note on Allport's "On knowing the meaning of words we are unable to report." *Quarterly Journal of Experimental Psychology*, 1978, *30*, 569–575.

Ellis, A. W., Miller, D., and Sin, G. Wernicke's aphasia and normal language processing: A case study in cognitive neuropsychology. *Cognition*, 1983.

Ellis, N. C. and Miles, T. R. A lexical encoding deficiency I: Experimental evidence. In G. Th. Pavlidis and T. R. Miles (Eds.), *Dyslexia Research and its Applications to Education*. London: John Wiley, 1981.

Flower, L. S. and Hayes, J. R. The dynamics of composing: Making plans and juggling constraints. In L. W. Gregg and E. R. Steinberg (Eds.), *Cognitive Processes in Writing*. Hillsdale, N.J.: Lawrence Erlbaum, 1980.

Forster, K. I. Priming and the effects of sentence and lexical contexts on naming time: Evidence for autonomous lexical processing. *Quarterly Journal of Experimental Psychology*, 1981, *33A*, 465–495.

Foss, D. J. and Hakes, D. T. *Psycholinguistics*. New York: Holt, Rinehart and Winston, 1978.

Frederiksen, C. H. and Dominic, J. F. (Eds.) *Writing: The Nature, Development, and Teaching of Written Communication. Vol. 2: Process, Development and Communication*. Hillsdale, N.J.: Lawrence Erlbaum, 1982.

Friedman, R. B. and Perlman, M. B. On the underlying causes of semantic paralexias in a patient with deep dyslexia. *Neuropsychologia*, 1983.

Frith, U. Unexpected spelling problems. In U. Frith (Ed.), *Cognitive Processes in Spelling*. London: Academic Press, 1980 (a).

Frith, U. (Ed.), *Cognitive Processes in Spelling*. London: Academic Press, 1980 (b).

Fromkin, V. and Rodman, R. *An Introduction to Language*. New York: Holt, Rinehart and Winston, 1974.

Funnell, E. Phonological processes in reading: New evidence from acquired dyslexia. *British Journal of Psychology*, 1983, *74*, 159–180.

Garrett, M. F. Production of speech: Observations from normal and pathological language use. In A. W. Ellis (Ed.), *Normality and Pathology in Cognitive Functions*. London: Academic Press, 1982.

Gelb, I. J. *A Study of Writing* (2nd ed.). Chicago: University of Chicago Press, 1963.

Gibson, E. J. and Levin, H. *The Psychology of Reading*. Cambridge, Mass.: MIT Press, 1975.

Glushko, R. J. The organization and activation of orthographic knowledge in reading aloud. *Journal of Experimental Psychology: Human Perception and Performance*, 1979, *5*, 674–691.

Golinkoff, R. M. Phonemic awareness skills and reading achievement. In F. Murray and J. J. Pikulski (Eds.), *The Acquisition of Reading*. Baltimore, Md.: University Park Press, 1978.

Goodman, K. S. Reading: A psycholinguistic guessing game. *Journal of the Reading Specialist*, 1967, *6*, 126–135.

Gough, P. B. One second of reading. In J. P. Kavanagh and I. G. Mattingly (Eds.), *Language by Ear and by Eye*. Cambridge, Mass.: MIT Press, 1972.

Gregg, L. W. and Steinberg, E. R. (Eds.), *Cognitive Processes in Writing*. Hillsdale, N.J.: Lawrence Erlbaum, 1980.

Halle, M. Some thoughts on spelling. In K. S. Goodman and J. T. Fleming (Eds.), *Psycholinguistics and the Teaching of Reading*. Newark, Del.: International Reading Association, 1969.

Hartley, J. (Ed.), *The Psychology of Written Communication*. London: Kogan Page, 1980.

Hatfield, F. M. and Patterson, K. E. Phonological spelling. *Quarterly Journal of Experimental Psychology*, 1983, *35A*, 451-468.

Hayes, J. R. and Flower, L. S. Identifying the organization of writing processes. In L. W. Gregg and E. R. Steinberg (Eds.), *Cognitive Processes in Writing*. Hillsdale, N.J.: Lawrence Erlbaum, 1980.

Healy, J. M. The enigma of hyperlexia. *Reading Research Quarterly*, 1982, *17*, 319-338.

Henderson, L. *Orthography and Word Recognition in Reading*. London: Academic Press, 1982.

Hermann, K. and Voldby, H. The morphology of handwriting in congenital word-blindness. *Acta Psychiatrica et Neurologica*, 1946, *21*, 349-363.

Hinshelwood, J. *Congenital Word Blindness*. London: H. K. Lewis, 1917.

Holmes, J. M. Dyslexia: A neurolinguistic study of traumatic and developmental disorders of reading. Unpublished Ph.D. thesis, University of Edinburgh, 1973.

Holmes, J. M. "Regression" and reading breakdown. In A. Caramazza and E. B. Zurif (Eds.), *Language Acquisition and Language Breakdown: Parallels and Divergences*. Baltimore: Johns Hopkins University Press, 1978.

Holmes, M. C. Investigation of reading readiness of first grade entrants. *Childhood Education*, 1928, *3*, 215-221.

Hornsby, B. and Miles, T. R. The effects of a dyslexia-centered teaching programme. *British Journal of Educational Psychology*, 1980, *50*, 236-242.

Hotopf, W. H. N. Slips of the pen. In U. Frith (Ed.), *Cognitive Processes in Spelling*. London: Academic Press, 1980.

Hughes, J. R. The electroencephalogram and reading disorders. In R. N. Malatesha and P. G. Aaron (Eds.), *Reading Disorders: Varieties and Treatments*. New York: Academic Press, 1982.

Huttenlocher, P. R. and Huttenlocher, J. A study of children with hyperlexia. *Neurology*, 1973, *23*, 1107-1116.

Ingram, T. T. S. The association of speech retardation and educational difficulties. *Proceedings of the Royal Society of Medicine*, 1963, *56*, 199-203.

Johnston, R. S. Developmental deep dyslexia. *Cortex*, 1983, *19*.

Jorm, A. F. The cognitive and neurological basis of developmental dyslexia: A theoretical framework and review. *Cognition*, 1979, *7*, 19-32.

Kavanagh, J. F. and Venezky, R. L. (Eds.), *Orthography, Reading and Dyslexia*. Baltimore: University Park Press, 1980.

Kay, J. and Marcel, T. One process not two in reading aloud: lexical analogies do the work of nonlexical rules. *Quarterly Journal of Experimental Psychology*, 1981, *33A*, 397-413.

Kertesz, A. *Aphasia and Associated Disorders: Taxonomy, Localization and Recovery*. New York: Grune and Stratton, 1979.

Kintsch, W. Semantic memory: A tutorial. In R. S. Nickerson (Ed.), *Attention and Performance, 8*. Hillsdale, N.J.: Lawrence Erlbaum, 1980.

Klatt, D. H. Lexical representations for speech production and perception. In T. Myers, J. Laver and J. Anderson (Eds.), *The Cognitive Representation of Speech*. Amsterdam: North-Holland, 1981.

Klein, R. Loss of written language due to dissolution of the phonetic structure of the word in brain abscess. *Journal of Mental Science*, 1951, *97*, 328-339.

Kolers, P. A. Reading and talking bilingually. *American Journal of Psychology*, 1966, *74*, 357-376.

Kress, G. *Learning to Write*. London: Routledge and Kegan Paul, 1982.

Leech, G., Deuchar, M., and Hoogenraad, R. *English Grammar for Today*. London: The Macmillan Press, 1982.

Levy, B. A. Vocalization and suppression effects in sentence memory. *Journal of Verbal Learning and Verbal Behaviour*, 1975, *14*, 304-316.

Levy, B. A.   Reading: Speech and meaning processes. *Journal of Verbal Learning and Verbal Behaviour*, 1977, *16*, 623–638.

Liberman, I., Liberman, A. M., Mattingly, I., and Shankweiler, D.   Orthography and the beginning reader. In J. F. Kavanagh and R. L. Venezky (Eds.), *Orthography, Reading and Dyslexia*. Baltimore: University Park Press, 1980.

Lieberman, P.   Some effects of semantic and grammatical context on the production and perception of speech. *Language and Speech*, 1963, *6*, 172–187.

Luria, A. R.   *Traumatic Aphasia*. The Hague: Mouton, 1970.

McClelland, J. L. and Rumelhart, D. E.   An interactive activation model of context effects in letter perception: Part 1. An account of basic findings. *Psychological Review*, 1981, *88*, 375–407.

Malatesha, R. N. and Aaron, P. G. (Eds.), *Reading Disorders: Varieties and Treatments*. New York: Academic Press, 1982.

Marcel, T.   Surface dyslexia and beginning reading: a revised hypothesis of the pronunciation of print and its impairments. In M. Coltheart, K. E. Patterson, and J. C. Marshall (Eds.), *Deep Dyslexia*. London: Routledge and Kegan Paul, 1980.

Marr, D.   Early processing of visual information. *Philosophical Transactions of the Royal Society of London, B*, 1976, *275*, 483–524.

Marsh, G., Friedman, M., Welch, V., and Desberg, P.   A cognitive-developmental theory of reading acquisition. In G. E. Mackinnon and T. G. Waller (Eds.), *Reading Research: Advances in Theory and Practice*. New York: Academic Press, 1981.

Marshall, J. C. and Newcombe, F.   Syntactic and semantic errors in paralexia. *Neuropsychologia*, 1966, *4*, 169–176.

Marshall, J. C. and Newcombe, F.   Patterns of paralexia: A psycholinguistic approach. *Journal of Psycholinguistic Research*, 1973, *2*, 175–199.

Marshall, J. C. and Newcombe, F.   The conceptual status of deep dyslexia: an historical perspective. In M. Coltheart, K. E. Patterson, and J. C. Marshall (Eds.), *Deep Dyslexia*. London: Routledge and Kegan Paul, 1980.

Marslen-Wilson, W. D.   Speech understanding as a psychological process. In J. C. Simon (Ed.), *Spoken Language Generation and Understanding*. Dortrecht: D. Reidel, 1980.

Masland, R. L.   Neurological aspects of dyslexia. In G. Th. Pavlidis and T. R. Miles (Eds.), *Dyslexia Research and its Applications to Education*. Chichester: John Wiley, 1981.

Mason, M. and Katz, L.   Visual processing of nonlinguistic strings: Redundancy effects and reading disability. *Journal of Experimental Psychology: General*, 1976, *105*, 338–348.

Meyer, D. E. and Schvaneveldt, R. W.   Facilitation in recognizing pairs of words: Evidence of a dependence between retrieval operations. *Journal of Experimental Psychology*, 1971, *90*, 227–234.

Miles, T. R.   *Dyslexia: The Pattern of Difficulties*. London: Granada, 1983.

Miles, T. R. and Ellis, N. C.   A lexical encoding deficiency II: Clinical observations. In G. Th. Pavlidis and T. R. Miles (Eds.), *Dyslexia Research and its Applications to Education*. Chichester: John Wiley, 1981.

Mitchell, D. C.   *The Process of Reading*. Chichester: J. Wiley, 1982.

Mitterer, J. O.   There are at least two kinds of poor readers: Whole-word poor readers and recoding poor readers. *Canadian Journal of Psychology*, 1982, *36*, 445–461.

Morais, J., Cary, L., Alegria, J., and Bertelson, P.   Does awareness of speech as a sequence of phones arise spontaneously? *Cognition*, 1979, *7*, 323–331.

Morton, J.   A preliminary function model for language behaviour. *International Audiology*, 1964, *3*, 216–225 (Reprinted in R. C. Oldfield and J. C. Marshall, Eds. *Language*. London: Penguin Books, 1968), (a).

Morton, J.   The effect of context on the visual duration threshold for words. *British Journal of Psychology*, 1964, *55*, 165–180 (b).

Morton, J.   A model for continuous language behaviour. *Language and Speech*, 1964, *7*, 40–70 (c).

Morton, J.   Interaction of information in word recognition. *Psychological Review*, 1969, *76*, 165–178.

Morton, J.   Word recognition. In J. Morton and J. C. Marshall (Eds.), *Psycholinguistic Series, Vol. 2*. London: Elek Science and Cambridge, Mass.: MIT Press, 1979 (a).

Morton, J.   Facilitation in word recognition: Experiments causing change in the logogen model. In P. A. Kolers, M. Wrolstad and H. Bouma (Eds.), *Processing of Visible Language, Vol. 1*. New York: Plenum, 1979 (b).

Morton, J.   The logogen model and orthographic structure. In U. Frith (Ed.), *Cognitive Processes in Spelling*. London: Academic Press, 1980.

Morton, J.   Disintegrating the lexicon: An information processing approach. In J. Mehler, E. C. T. Walker and M. Garrett (Eds.), *Perspectives on Mental Representation*. Hillsdale, N.J.: Lawrence Erlbaum, 1982.

Morton, J. and Patterson, K. E.   A new attempt at an interpretation, or, an attempt at a new interpretation. In M. Coltheart, K. E. Patterson and J. C. Marshall (Eds.), *Deep Dyslexia*. London: Routledge and Kegan Paul, 1980.

Murrell, G. and Morton, J.   Word recognition and morphemic structure. *Journal of Experimental Psychology*, 1974, *102*, 963–968.

Naidoo, S.   Teaching methods and their rationale. In G. Th. Pavlidis and T. R. Miles (Eds.), *Dyslexia Research and its Applications to Education*. New York: John Wiley, 1981.

Newcombe, F. and Marshall, J. C.   Transcoding and lexical stabilization in deep dyslexia. In M. Coltheart, K. E. Patterson, and J. C. Marshall (Eds.), *Deep Dyslexia*. London: Routledge and Kegan Paul, 1980.

Newcombe, F. and Marshall, J. C.   On psycholinguistic classifications of the acquired dyslexias. *Bulletin of the Orton Society*, 1981, *31*, 29–46.

Newton, M. and Wilsher, C.   *Dyslexia: The Aston Perspective*. Birmingham: University of Aston, 1979.

Olson, D. R.   From utterance to text: The bias of language in speech and writing. *Harvard Educational Review*, 1977, *47*, 257–281.

O'Regan, K.   Saccade size control in reading: Evidence for the linguistic control hypothesis. *Perception and Psychophysics*, 1979, *25*, 501–509.

Orton, S. T.   Special disability in spelling. *Bulletin of the Neurological Clinic*, 1931, *1*, 159–192.

Orton, S. T.   *Reading, Writing and Speech Problems in Children*. New York: Norton, 1937.

Patterson, K. E.   What's right with 'deep' dyslexics. *Brain and Language*, 1979, *8*, 111–129.

Patterson, K. E.   Neuropsychological approaches to the study of reading. *British Journal of Psychology*, 1981, *72*, 151–174.

Patterson, K. E.   The relation between reading and phonological coding: Further neuropsychological observations. In A. W. Ellis (Ed.), *Normality and Pathology in Cognitive Functions*. London: Academic Press, 1982.

Patterson, K. and Kay, J.   Letter-by-letter reading: Psychological descriptions of a neurological syndrome. *Quarterly Journal of Experimental Psychology*, 1982, *34A*, 411–441.

Pavlidis, G. Th.   Sequencing, eye movements and the early objective diagnosis of dyslexia. In G. Th. Pavlidis and T. R. Miles (Eds.), *Dyslexia Research and its Applications to Education*. Chichester: John Wiley, 1981.

Pavlidis, G. Th.   Erratic sequential eye movements in dyslexics: comments and reply to Stanley *et al. British Journal of Psychology*, 1983, *74*, 189–193.

Pavlidis, G. Th. and Miles, T. R. (Eds.), *Dyslexia Research and its Applications to Education*. Chichester: John Wiley, 1981.

Perfetti, C. A., Goldman, S. R., and Hogaboam, T. W.   Reading skill and the identification of words in discourse context. *Memory and Cognition*, 1979, *4*, 273-282.

Perfetti, C. A. and Roth, S.   Some of the interactive processes in reading and their role in reading skill. In A. M. Lesgold and C. Perfetti (Eds.), *Interactive Processes in Reading*. Hillsdale, N.J.: Lawrence Erlbaum, 1981.

Pintner, R.   Inner speech during silent reading. *Psychological Review*, 1913, *20*, 129-153.

Pirozzolo, F. J. and Hansch, E. C.   The neurobiology of developmental reading disorders. In R. N. Malatesha and P. G. Aaron (Eds.), *Reading Disorders: Varieties and Treatments*. New York: Academic Press, 1982.

Pirozzolo, F. J. and Wittrock, M. C. (Eds.),   *Neuropsychological and Cognitive Processes in Reading*. New York: Academic Press, 1981.

Plessas, G. P.   Children's errors in spelling homonyms. *Elementary School Journal*, 1963, *64*, 163-168.

Potter, M. C. and Faulconer, B. A.   Time to understand pictures and words. *Nature (London)*, 1975, *253*, 437-438.

Ratcliff, G. and Newcombe, F.   Object recognition: some deductions from the clinical evidence. In A. W. Ellis (Ed.), *Normality and Pathology in Cognitive Functions*. London: Academic Press, 1982.

Rayner, K.   Eye movements in reading and information processing. *Psychological Bulletin*, 1978, *85*, 618-660.

Rayner, K.   Visual selective attention in reading and search: A tutorial review. In H. Bouma and D. Bowhuis (Eds.), *Attention and Performance 10*. Hillsdale, N.J.: Lawrence Erlbaum, 1983.

Rayner, K., Well, A. D., and Pollatsek, A.   Asymmetry of the effective visual field in reading. *Perception and Psychophysics*, 1980, *27*, 537-544.

Read, C.   Pre-school children's knowledge of English phonology. *Harvard Educational Review*, 1971, *41*, 1-34.

Richman, L. C. and Kitchell, M. M.   Hyperlexia as a variant of developmental language disorder. *Brain and Language*, 1981, *12*, 203-212.

Robinson, P., Beresford, R., and Dodd, B.   Spelling errors made by phonologically disordered children. *Bulletin of the Simplified Spelling Society*, 1982, *22*, 19-20.

Rosati, G. and Bastiani, P. de.   Pure agraphia: a discrete form of aphasia. *Journal of Neurology, Neurosurgery and Psychiatry*, 1979, *42*, 266-269.

Rozin, P. and Gleitman, L. R.   The structure and acquisition of reading II: The reading process and the acquisition of the alphabetic principle. In A. S. Reber and D. L. Scarborough (Eds.), *Towards a Psychology of Reading*. Hillsdale, N.J.: Lawrence Erlbaum, 1977.

Rubenstein, H., Lewis, S. S., and Rubenstein, M. A.   Evidence for phonemic recording in visual word recognition. *Journal of Verbal Learning and Verbal Behaviour*, 1971, *10*, 645-657.

Rugel, R. P.   WISC subtest scores of disabled readers. *Journal of Learning Disabilities*, 1974, *7*, 57-64.

Rumelhart, D. E. and McClelland, J. L.   Interactive processing through spreading activation. In A. M. Lesgold and C. A. Perfetti (Eds.), *Interactive Processes in Reading*. Hillsdale, N.J.: Lawrence Erlbaum, 1981.

Rumelhart, D. E. and McClelland, J. L.   An interactive model of context effects in letter perception: Part 2. The contextual enhancement effect and some tests and extensions of the model. *Psychological Review*, 1982, *89*, 60-94.

Saffran, E. M.   Neuropsychological approaches to the study of language. *British Journal of Psychology*, 1982, *73*, 317-337.

Saffran, E. M., Bogyo, L. C., Schwartz, M. F. and Marin, O. S. M.   Does deep dyslexia reflect right-hemisphere reading? In M. Coltheart, K. E. Patterson, and J. C. Marshall (Eds.), *Deep Dyslexia*. London: Routledge and Kegan Paul, 1980.

Sanford, A. J. and Garrod, S. C.   *Understanding Written Language: Explorations in Comprehension Beyond the Sentence*. Chichester: J. Wiley, 1981.

Satz, P. and Morris, R.   Learning disability subtypes: A review. In F. J. Pirozzolo and M. C. Wittrock (Eds.), *Neuropsychological and Cognitive Processes in Reading*. New York: Academic Press, 1981.

Schwartz, M. F., Marin, O. S. M., and Saffran, E. M.   Dissociations of language function in dementia: A case study. *Brain and Language*, 1979, *7*, 277-306.

Schwartz, M. F., Saffran, E. M., and Marin, O. S. M.   Fractionating the reading process in dementia: Evidence for word-specific print-to-sound associations. In M. Coltheart, K. E. Patterson and J. C. Marshall (Eds.), *Deep Dyslexia*. London: Routledge and Kegan Paul, 1980.

Seymour, P. H. K.   *Human Visual Cognition*. West Drayton: Collier Macmillan, 1979.

Seymour, P. H. K. and Porpodas, C. D.   Lexical and non-lexical processing of spelling in developmental dyslexia. In U. Frith (Ed.), *Cognitive Processes in Spelling*. London: Academic Press, 1980.

Shallice, T.   Phonological agraphia and the lexical route in writing. *Brain*, 1981, *104*, 413-429.

Shallice, T., Warrington, E. K. and McCarthy, R.   Reading without semantics. *Quarterly Journal of Experimental Psychology*, 1983, *35A.*, 111-138.

Shallice, T. and Warrington, E. K.   Single and multiple component central dyslexic syndromes. In M. Coltheart, K. E. Patterson and J. C. Marshall (Eds.), *Deep Dyslexia*. London: Routledge and Kegan Paul, 1980.

Shallice, T., Warrington, E. K. and McCarthy, R.   Reading without semantics. *Quarterly Journal of Experimental Psychology*, 1983, *35A*.

Silberberg, N. E. and Silberberg, M. C.   Case histories in hyperlexia. *Journal of School Psychology*, 1968, *7*, 3-7.

Simpson, J. M.   Reading errors in nine-year-old children in comparison with developmental surface dyslexic. Unpublished undergraduate dissertation, Department of Psychology, University of Lancaster, 1983.

Sloboda, J.   Visual imagery and individual differences in spelling. In U. Frith (Ed.), *Cognitive Processes in Spelling*. London: Academic Press, 1980.

Slowiaczek, M. L. and Clifton, C.   Subvocalisation and reading for meaning. *Journal of Verbal Learning and Verbal Behaviour*, 1980, *19*, 573-582,

Snowling, M. J.   The development of grapheme-phoneme correspondences in normal and dyslexic readers. *Journal of Experimental Child Psychology*, 1980, *29*, 294-305.

Snowling, M. J.   Phonemic deficits in developmental dyslexia. *Psychological Research*, 1981, *43*, 219-234.

Sokolov, A. N.   *Inner Speech and Thought*. New York: Plenum, 1972.

Solomons, L. M. and Stein, G.   Normal motor automatisms. *Psychological Review*, 1896, *3*, 492-512.

Søvik, N.   *Developmental Cybernetic of Handwriting and Graphic Behaviour*. Oslo: Universitetsforlaget, 1975.

Spelke, E., Hirst, W. and Neisser, U.   Skills of divided attention. *Cognition*, 1976, *4*, 215-230.

Springer, S. P. and Deutsch, G.   *Left Brain, Right Brain*. San Francisco: W. H. Freeman, 1981.

Stanley, G.   Eye movements in dyslexic children. In G. Stanley and K. W. Walsh (Eds.), *Brain Impairment: Proceedings of the 1977 Brain Impairment Workshop*. Victoria: The Dominion Press, 1978.

Stanley, G., Smith, G. A., and Howell, E. A.   Eye movements and sequential tracking in dyslexic and control children. *British Journal of Psychology*, 1983a, *74*, 181-187.

Stanley, G., Smith, G. A., and Howell, E. A.   Eye movements in dyslexic children: Comments on Pavlidis' reply. *British Journal of Psychology*, 1983b, *74*, 195-197.

Stanovich, K. E.   Attentional and automatic context effects in reading. In A. M. Lesgold and C. Perfetti (Eds.), *Interactive Processes in Reading*. Hillsdale, N.J.: Lawrence Erlbaum, 1981.

Stubbs, M.   *Language and Literacy: The Sociolinguistics of Reading and Writing*. London: Routledge and Kegan Paul, 1980.

Temple, C. M. and Marshall, J. C.   A case study of developmental phonological dyslexia. *British Journal of Psychology*, 1983, *74*.

Tenney, Y. J.   Visual factors in spelling. In U. Frith (Ed.), *Cognitive Processes in Spelling*. London: Academic Press, 1980.

Thomassen, A. J. W. M. and Teulings, H.-L. H. M.   The development of directional preference in writing movements. *Visible Language*, 1979, *13*, 299-313.

Thomson, M. E.   The assessment of children with specific reading difficulties (dyslexia) using the British Ability Scales. *British Journal of Psychology*, 1982, *73*, 461-478.

Torgeson, J. K. and Houck, D. G.   Processing deficiencies of learning-disabled children who perform poorly on the digit span test. *Journal of Educational Psychology*, 1980, *72*, 141-160.

Tulving, E. and Gold, C.   Stimulus information and contextual information as determinants of tachistoscopic recognition of words. *Journal of Experimental Psychology*, 1963, *66*, 319-327.

Valenstein, E. and Heilman, K. M.   Apraxic agraphia with neglect-induced paragraphia. *Archives of Neurology*, 1979, *36*, 506-508.

Vellutino, F. R.   *Dyslexia: Theory and Research*. Cambridge, Mass.: MIT Press, 1979.

Vernon, M. D.   Variability in reading retardation. *British Journal of Psychology*, 1979, *70*, 7-16.

Warren, C. and Morton, J.   The effects of priming on picture recognition. *British Journal of Psychology*, 1982, *73*, 117-130.

Warrington, E. K.   The incidence of verbal disability associated with reading retardation. *Neuropsychologia*, 1967, *5*, 175-179.

Warrington, E. K. and Shallice, T.   Word-form dyslexia. *Brain*, 1980, *103*, 99-112.

Wason, P. C.   Specific thoughts on the writing process. In L. W. Gregg and E. R. Steinberg (Eds.), *Cognitive Processes in Writing*. Hillsdale, N.J.: Lawrence Erlbaum, 1980.

Weber, R.-M.   The study of oral reading errors: A survey of the literature. *Reading Research Quarterly*, 1968, *4*, 96-119.

Wells, F. L.   Linguistic lapses. In J. McK. Cattell and F. J. E. Woodbridge (Eds.), *Archives of Philosophy, Psychology and Scientific Methods No. 6*. New York: Science Press, 1906.

Wernicke, C.   *Der Aphasische Symptomencomplex*. Breslau: Cohn and Weigart, 1874 (Translated in G. H. Eggert, *Wernicke's Works on Aphasia*. The Hague: Mouton, 1977).

West, R. F. and Stanovich, K. D.   Automatic contextual facilitation in readers of three ages. *Child Development*, 1978, *49*, 717-727.

Wing, A. M. and Baddeley, A. D.   Spelling errors in handwriting: A corpus and a distributional analysis. In U. Frith (Ed.), *Cognitive Processes in Spelling*. London: Academic Press, 1980.

Winograd, T.   *Understanding Natural Language*. New York: Academic Press, 1972.

Zurif, E. G. and Carson, G.   Dyslexia in relation to cerebral dominance and temporal analysis. *Neuropsychologia*, 1970, *8*, 351-361.

Author Index

140

Diringer, D., 3
Doctor, E. A., 99
Dodd, B., 98
Dominic, J. F., 96
Douse, T. le M., 68
Downing, J., 99, 103

Ehrlich, S. F., 93
Eldridge, M., 58
Elliott, D. E., 97
Ellis, A. W., 26, 31, 45, 68, 70, 75, 79, 80, 113, 114
Ellis, N. C., 108, 109, 110, 111, 113

Faulconer, B. A., 28
Flower, L. S., 61, 62
Forster, K. I., 54
Foss, D. J., 21, 51
Frederiksen, C. H., 96
Friedman, M., 87, 88, 89, 90, 93, 97, 103, 117
Friedman, R. B., 43
Frith, U., 60, 107, 126
Fromkin, V., 3
Funnell, E., 15, 37, 81

Garrett, M. F., 27
Garrod, S. C., 51, 52
Gelb, I. J., 1, 3
Gentner, D., 62
Gibson, E., 56
Gipson, P., 31
Gleitman, L. R., 101
Glucksberg, S., 52
Glushko, R. J., 29, 30, 90
Gold, C., 53, 54
Goldman, S. R., 93
Golinkoff, R. M., 101
Goodman, K. S., 92, 93
Gough, P. B., 15
Gregg, L. W., 60

Hakes, D. T., 21, 51
Halle, M., 7, 8
Hansch, E. E., 111
Hartley, J., 60
Hatfield, F. M., 64, 76, 77, 98
Hayes, J. R., 61, 62
Healy, J. M., 120
Heilman, K. M., 78, 80
Henderson, L., 15, 39, 46, 54
Hermann, K., 127

Hinshelwood, J., 107, 112, 118, 121
Hirst, W., 82
Hogaboam, T. W., 93
Holmes, J. M., 40, 114, 115
Holmes, M. C., 100
Hoogenraad, R., 61
Hornsby, B., 127
Hotopf, W. H. N., 68, 70
Houck, D. G., 110, 111
Howell, E. A., 109
Hughes, J. R., 111
Huttenlocher, J., 119, 120
Huttenlocher, P. R., 119, 120

Ingram, T. T. S., 110, 115

Javal, 49
Johnston, R. S., 114
Jonasson, J. T., 91
Jorm, A. F., 111, 112, 115

Katz, L., 108
Kavanagh, J. F., 107
Kay, J., 30, 44, 46, 70, 83, 84, 90
Kellman, P., 75
Kenyon, R. V., 109
Kerr, J., 107
Kertesz, A., 35, 65, 66
Kintsch, W., 21
Kitchell, M. M., 120
Klatt, D. H., 12
Klein, R., 78
Kolers, P. A., 56
Kress, G., 96

Leech, G., 61
Leong, C. K., 103
Levin, H., 56
Levy, B. A., 58
Lewis, S. S., 15
Lewis, V. J., 58, 113
Liberman, A. M., 101
Liberman, I., 101
Lieberman, P., 55
Luria, A. R, 63, 64

McCarthy, R., 46
McClelland, J. L., 17, 21, 25, 34
Malatesha, R. N., 107, 124
Marcel, A. J., 30, 39, 46, 70, 90, 92
Marin, O. S. M., 28, 37, 44, 46, 120
Marr, D., 44

Voldby, H., 127

Warren, C., 28
Warrington, E. K., 36, 37, 39, 43, 44, 46, 83, 84, 111
Wason, P. C., 61
Weber, R.-M., 92
Welch, V., 87, 88, 89 90, 93, 97, 103, 117
Well, A. D., 49
Wells, F. L., 68, 79, 113

Wernicke, C., 15, 35
West, R. F., 93
Wilf, J. F., 75
Wilsher, C., 110
Wing, A. M., 68, 74
Winograd, T., 52
Witrock, M. C., 107

Zurif, E. G., 116

Subject Index

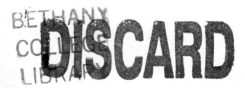